Perspectives in Health Care

Perspectives in Health Care

WX 120

First published 1997 by
MACMILLAN PRESS LTD
Houndmills, Basingstoke, Hampshire RG21 6XS
and London
Companies and representatives
throughout the world

ISBN 0–333–61465–8

A catalogue record for this book is available
from the British Library.

This book is printed on paper suitable for recycling and
made from fully managed and sustained forest sources.

10   9   8   7   6   5   4   3   2   1
07   06   05   04   03   02   01   00   99   98

Copy-edited and typeset by Povey–Edmondson
Tavistock and Rochdale, England

Printed in Hong Kong

For Rebecca, Alice and Ben;
Holly and Tom

Contents

Foreword   viii
List of Contributors   x
Introduction   xi

1 Perspectives   1
   Yvonne Bradshaw

2 Policy Processes   23
   Nancy North

3 Health Care Models and Welfare Themes   47
   Ian Kendall

4 Individual Responsibility or Citizen Rights?   67
   Ian Kendall and Graham Moon

5 Managers and Professionals   84
   Rosemary Gillespie

6 Markets and Choice   110
   Graham Moon

7 Consumers, Service Users or Citizens?   130
   Nancy North

8 Market Testing, Market Failure: Health Service
   Privatisation in Theory and Practice, 1979–96   150
   John Mohan

9 Conclusion   170
   Nancy North and Yvonne Bradshaw

Index   187

Foreword

When Iain Macleod observed in 1958 that 'The National Health Service, with the exception of recurring spasms about charges, is out of party politics', few would have disagreed that the debate about principles and values was behind us (quoted in R. Klein, *The New Politics of the NHS*, Longman, 1995, p. 29). After intense struggle to establish the NHS and a decade of structural reform, it did appear, by the late 1950s, that the fundamental questions about how to finance and organise the new national service had all been resolved. A broader analysis of public policies for health over the last century, however, demonstrates that major debates about ideology and practice both preceded the relative calm of the 1950s and persist to the present day. Although the foreign observer has come to see the British NHS as an immovable rock, around which the turbulent waters of social, economic and political change may be swirling, the recent threats to its funding and structure cast doubt upon its stability and future. The chapters in this book illustrate clearly that the NHS, as conceived in 1948, cannot be taken for granted and that many critical challenges remain.

What is striking, in the discussion which follows, is the endurance in British health policy of some traditional themes and questions. Who should provide health care (families or the state, the individual or the collective, the local authority or the health service)? How should it be organised (through the market or the state, locally or centrally)? Who should determine its character (clinicians, users, managers or politicians)? How can it be funded (through taxation, insurance or charges)? And according to what principles should it be distributed (equity, equality, desert, clinical need, prognosis, ability to pay)? As the authors demonstrate, few, if any, of these questions can be regarded as answered for all time. Although there may be some doubt about the lasting impact of the post-1979 NHS 'reforms', over the longer term the real challenges which they posed to post-war social democratic welfare values cannot be overlooked.

As this book shows, the further we move away from some of the 'great events' in British health policy (the introduction of national insurance, the birth of the NHS, the creation of an internal market), the more we are able to analyse these developments with clarity. Changes which were described, in their day, as 'inevitable developments' or 'rational responses' to new circumstances can, with hindsight, be understood as the outcome of complex social processes which were neither inevitable not rational. The strength of this book lies in its interweaving of theoretical insight, analytical perspective and historical fact. All these elements are central to our understanding of health policy in the past and its prospects in the future.

JOAN HIGGINS
Professor of Health Policy
University of Manchester

List of Contributors

Yvonne Bradshaw is Lecturer in Social Policy at the University of Portsmouth. Her main research interests are in social policy and administration and social security policies. Previous publications have focused on the interface between health care and the criminal justice system.

Rosemary Gillespie is Lecturer in Sociology at the University of Portsmouth. She has published in the area of women and the body and is currently researching voluntary childlessness and women.

Ian Kendall is Professor of Social Policy at the University of Portsmouth. He has written on several aspects of health policy with both Graham Moon and John Carrier, including community care, complaints procedures and mental health services.

John Mohan is Reader in Geography, University of Portsmouth. He is the author of *A National Health Service? The Restructuring of Health Care in Britain since 1979* (Macmillan), editor of *The Political Geography of Contemporary Britain* (Macmillan) and the author of numerous articles and book chapters on health care policy. He is currently researching the historical geography of the British voluntary hospital system and the rise and fall of regionalism and regional planning of the hospital services.

Graham Moon is Professor of Health Services Research at the University of Portsmouth. He has research interests in the geography of health-related behaviour in medico-legal studies and in health policy reform with particular reference to primary care and to developments in East–Central Europe.

Nancy North is Lecturer in Health Policy at the University of Portsmouth. Previous publications have focused on internal markets and professional and consumer interests. Her current research interests are in health care commissioning, consumerism and primary health care.

Introduction

The National Health Service, together with all public services, has come under intense scrutiny and has been judged, by Conservative governments since 1979, as inefficient, wasteful and unresponsive to the needs of consumers. There are many aspects to the Conservatives' reform agenda for the health service, as the following chapters identify, but the general thrust of reform has been the pursuit of better value for (public) money within a quasi-market framework.

The principles which had underpinned the post-war welfare consensus came under sustained attack after the general election of 1979. The language of value for money, choice and self-help superseded that of equality, universalism and state provision. The health service was portrayed as a bureaucratised monopoly which was profligate in its use of taxpayers' money, with little interest in meeting the genuine needs of patients.

Evaluation and analysis of health care policy takes many forms and the way in which the New Right-influenced Conservative governments approach this will differ from that of advocates of alternative, competing perspectives. The differences between perspectives, the problems they highlight and the concomitant policy proposals are the themes pursued in Chapter 1 of this volume. Policy making is not a straightforward process of decision making and implementation. There are many complexities involved in this process and, as Chapter 2 demonstrates, a range of theories about how this process takes place. Even when a decision on policy has been reached, this can be changed during the process of implementation, a factor which is also discussed within this chapter. What health care policy should achieve, the way it should be provided and funded, lead to different models of health care provision being advocated. These models of health care, the way in which one model has been superseded by another in the past and the implications of this form the substance of Chapter 3.

After the initial three chapters outlining different ways of analysing health care, the models associated with different theoretical perspectives, and competing explanations of policy making, the following chapters focus on a number of themes within the debate about the provision of health care.

In Chapter 4, Ian Kendall and Graham Moon explore the tensions between individualist and collectivist approaches to welfare provision. They point out that in both historical and contemporary contexts there is no automatic association between the political right and individualism and the political left and collectivism. The chapter ends with the suggestion that, if society accepts the principle that everyone should have a reasonable standard of health care, there is a compelling case for maintaining a National Health Service. Rosemary Gillespie, in Chapter 5, explores the way in which professionals emerged as powerful occupational groups in the post-war period, able to attain both social status and high economic rewards. This power and prestige has been challenged by the move to implement market principles within the provision of health care. The discussion within this chapter covers a number of policy initiatives which have arguably had the effect of constraining this power and ends by suggesting that we have witnessed the rise of a new powerful occupational group, that of the professional manager. The focus on market principles is continued in Chapter 6 where Graham Moon provides a discussion of the systematic reform of British health care policy during the 1980s and 1990s. Beginning with a discussion of the market, this chapter moves on to discuss the continued importance of need within health policy. These opening theoretical issues are related to the practicalities of reform where most appropriate and the significance of the reforms that have taken place is evaluated towards the end of the chapter.

Consumerism and political participation are explored in Chapter 7. Nancy North examines both historic and contemporary evidence about the mechanisms by which lay groups and individuals can express their preferences and opinions. In doing so the author considers the extent to which the recent reforms have produced a health service more responsive to lay concerns and discusses the difficulties of mediating competing claims. Privatisation both in theory and in practice forms the major theme of Chapter 8. In this chapter, John Mohan offers a carefully considered account of the theoretical bases of privatisation and the rationale by which policies

have been explained and justified. This chapter ends with a consideration of the constraints on further privatisation taking place
within the National Health Service in the foreseeable future. The
final chapter in this collection acts as a summary of the main themes
of the book as well as indicating that changes within the health care
system and issues of concern to UK policy makers are not unique to
the UK.

The chapters in this book can be read individually and, while
certain themes and perspectives are addressed in several chapters,
there is no attempt to produce an integrated reader on health care
policy. Each chapter addresses a certain theme or issue concerned
with health care and applies some of the theoretical perspectives and
models in Chapters 1–3 to these themes or issues.

We hope you find the book stimulating and that it provides some
useful tools for explaining, analysing and evaluating the changes that
have taken place in health care policy in the post war period and, in
particular, the years of Conservative government.

Yvonne Bradshaw
Nancy North

1

Perspectives

Yvonne Bradshaw

This chapter provides a brief introduction to some of the major theoretical perspectives which have been used to analyse health policies and practice. The brevity with which each perspective is described is intended to provide a succinct but adequate foundation on which a more detailed analysis of health care provision will be built in subsequent chapters. Each perspective offers a distinctive approach to the analysis of policies and practice and a concomitant prescription for the future direction both should take. Adherence to one, rather than another, theoretical perspective determines not only the relative importance attached to specific issues, but also the evidence selected for analysis. For example, adopting a feminist perspective means that explaining women's experience of and treatment within the health system, is an issue of primary importance. Gender is used by feminists as a primary explanatory concept and evidence is therefore selected which exemplifies the different and unequal treatment of women and men within the health care system.

There are a number of different ways in which the major perspectives referred to in this chapter could have been labelled. I have chosen to use the terms 'social democratic', 'New Right', 'feminist', 'Marxist' and 'welfare pluralist' as these seem to be the most valuable in terms of analysing health care policy and provision. In addition, an anti-racist approach to the analysis of health care provision, while not perhaps as developed as the other approaches (Williams, 1989), is also discussed. Within these primary ideologies or perspectives there are a number of groupings and strands which exhibit differences in focus and explanation, but have sufficient concerns in common to be classified within the main perspective. Again feminism provides a good, though not unique, example of this. Within the umbrella category of feminism, there are a range of approaches and strands which include, for example, liberal feminists, socialist feminists, radical feminists and black feminists. The differing explanations offered for women's unequal position and the degree of oppression they experience exemplify a significant divide or even disunity amongst feminists. What unites feminists, however, is the belief that 'an analysis of the position of women is not marginal but central to a true understanding of the nature of the Welfare State' (Wilson, 1977: 39).

The social democratic perspective provides another example of an umbrella term which incorporates a range of approaches, amongst which there are differences in focus and emphases. What draws these various approaches together, though not always unproblematically, is firstly a recognition that unfettered markets can produce levels of inequality which are viewed as socially unjust and inefficient and secondly, a belief in the value of collective action and planning via the state, as a means of meeting social needs.

All the perspectives discussed in this and subsequent chapters not only offer a critical evaluation of health policies and health care practice, but are also either implicitly or explicitly prescriptive. This leads each perspective to advocate a particular model of health care provision, some of which are discussed in more detail in Chapter 3. The role played by the state in the provision of welfare is of vital importance in both the critiques and policy prescriptions of these perspectives. Explanations about what is and what should be the role of the state are therefore integral to the debates about the best means of providing health care.

Social Democratic Perspective

The aim of those working from within a social democratic perspective was, and arguably still is, to create a more equal, socially just and democratic society within the existing capitalist system. In seeking to engineer this ideal society, social democrats have criticised the operation of unfettered markets and many of the subsequent dis-tributional outcomes as unjust, in that they produce unacceptable levels of inequality. This critique has led advocates of this perspective, some more reluctantly than others, to advocate collectively funded and provided welfare services and an active role for the state in the provision and distribution of these services.

According to social democrats, free market provision and distribution can lead to a number of problems. It is contended that unregulated markets can be economically inefficient and prevent the creation of a socially just society. Whilst markets can provide certain benefits, they are also believed to encourage self-interest and greed, lead to concentrations of economic power and political power and thus to the perpetuation of unacceptable inequalities. Many of the inequalities resulting from market distribution are viewed as both wasteful in terms of human talent (Crosland, 1956) and socially unjust. It is not suggested that state provision should totally displace market provision, even in the sphere of welfare. Rather the aim is that, in the main, socially important goods such as health care, which are viewed as qualitatively different from market goods, be provided collectively via the state and not left to the inequitable outcomes of impersonal market forces.

The social democratic perspective was at its most dominant in the period after the Second World War, a period during which the welfare state developed and expanded. The influence of this perspective can be detected in many of the social policies pursued in this post-war period, not least of which were the policies pursued in the field of health. In reviewing the analysis of health care provision offered by a social democratic perspective, the work of Richard Titmuss, Thomas Marshall, Anthony Crosland and, at a later date, that of Peter Townsend, provides a good beginning.

It was during the Second World War that plans began to be made for the type of society which was to come into being at the end of the war. This post-war society was to be based on the same guiding principles that had influenced the emergency services during the war, that is the pooling of resources and the sharing of risks (Marshall, 1975: 83). As Titmuss pointed out, these principles were not 'always practicable nor always applied; but they were the guiding principles' (cited in Marshall, 1975).

The Beveridge Report of 1942 is often cited as a document which had a momentous effect on post-war social policy. Beveridge, while certainly a social reformer, has also been labelled as a 'reluctant collectivist' in that he initially believed market provision to be preferable to state provision, in terms of both efficiency and the promotion of individual freedom. Beveridge, however, came to recognise that the unfettered market was producing unacceptable social inequalities and disadvantages and accepted, albeit reluctantly, the need for state intervention. The Beveridge Report, while mainly concerned with providing effective social security to counteract the problem of 'want', also recognised the concomitant need to tackle other related problems, one of which was 'disease'. This Report paved the way for action in the field of health care in the post-war period by recommending that provision be made for 'comprehensive health and rehabilitation services' (Beveridge, 1942 Appendix F: 287).

The principles on which post-war health care provision was based clearly reflect the social democratic influence. These principles were, firstly, that the service should be financed by taxation and contributions, paid while people were well, rather than charging people for medical services when the need arose; secondly, that the financial cost of providing the service should be borne by the whole community; and thirdly, that the service should be national in terms of providing the same high quality service across the whole country (Marshall, 1975: 137).

According to Richard Titmuss (1963), the fundamental belief that no one should go without health care because they could not pay led directly to the further principle of comprehensiveness. Acceptance of the principle of comprehensiveness created 'a new public responsibility; to make it in future somebody's clear duty to see that all medical facilities are available to all people'(HMSO, 1944: 47). These principles, together with the failure of the market to produce an efficient or sufficient health care system which provided everyone with equal access to medical care, led to the state taking an active role in planning and delivering a tax-funded national health care service (Titmuss, 1963)

The National Health Service (NHS), inaugurated in July 1948, therefore reflected the social democratic principles of pooling of resources and sharing risks. Collectively everyone pays for the health system as a whole; what an individual citizen has a right to receive is related, not to their contribution, even if they have made no contribution at all, but to their status as a citizen.

Whilst Titmuss and other writers from within this social democratic perspective were critical of some of the outcomes of health policies pursued during the post-war period, they staunchly defended the principles of the NHS from attacks from the New Right (see Titmuss, 1976) and from the Marxist left (see Crosland, 1956).

Titmuss supported universal state provision on both economic and moral grounds. He pointed out that New Right commentators were wrong to believe that economic growth alone would ensure that poverty and inequality would cease to be a problem. More importantly Titmuss argued that the welfare state was concerned not only with tackling poverty and disadvantage, but also with promoting social justice. He argued that part of the role of the welfare state was to compensate people for 'diswelfare' created by economic progress, for example unemployment created by technological advance, or ill-health caused by industrialisation and pollution. The market, if left to its own devices, would not provide for those affected by economic changes (Titmuss, 1976).

From this perspective, health care is not simply another consumer good which can be effectively provided via the market. Titmuss listed 13 characteristics or factors which differentiate health care from consumer goods, of which he claimed the most important were the uncertainty and unpredictability involved in the need for health care provision (Titmuss, 1976: 143–5).

Welfare policies were advocated not only as an important means of reducing the scale of inequality, but also as a potentially positive contribution to economic growth. Moreover, economic growth was viewed as an important and necessary prerequisite for implementing the redistributive welfare policies necessary to tackle inequalities. Crosland (1956) pointed out that any attempt to implement redistributive policies needed an expanding economy if social antagonism was to be avoided. If the absolute position of the better off was maintained through economic growth, Crosland believed these groups would accept the change in their relative position brought about by redistribution. According to advocates of this perspective, the central state was the only institution in society with the ability rationally to organise welfare provision and redistribute resources in a manner which would bring about the desired reduction in inequalities and promotion of social justice and democracy.

The social democratic perspective provides both a rationale for state provision of welfare and a justification for universal rather than selective access to services. While the problems of an unfettered market mechanism were recognised, there was never any attempt to displace private or commercial provision totally. Commercial provision continued alongside state-provided education, health care and social insurance. An expanding economy in the post-war period resulted in full or nearly full employment, which not only provided the revenue for welfare expenditure but also reduced the need for some welfare services. It was within such economic circumstances that social democrats optimistically advocated centrally organised, redistributive policies which it was assumed would engineer a more equal, socially just society and health care system within it.

In the 1940s it was believed that one of the main barriers to access to health care was price. Thus making health care free to all at the point of use and ensuring the best possible standards affordable were provided nationally was viewed as the answer to inequality and social injustice. Accordingly social democrats advocated what has been referred to as a universal citizenship model of health care provision (see Chapter 3). Universality rather than selectivity in welfare provision was also important in that the former not only promoted a sense of community and reciprocity but also helped to maintain higher standards of service provision (Titmuss, 1976).

Simply removing the price barrier did not reduce inequalities however, as later research clearly indicated (see Abel-Smith and Townsend 1965; Black Report 1980). Moreover, as discussed in Chapters 5 and 6, the NHS was virtually a monopoly service, with all the concomitant problems of monopoly provision. The doctors working within the system exercised a great deal of power with little effective democratic accountability. This monopolistic provision, the power of the medical profession and their paternalistic approach to patients, together with the continuation of inequalities, were all subsequently the focus of criticism. The following perspectives were influential in generating a critique of the welfare state which encompasses the NHS.

New Right Perspective

The New Right perspective includes two main strands of thought, which have been labelled in various ways. The first is the economic liberal strand with its ideological commitment to market provision. According to this group of theorists, the market is believed to be, not only the most efficient means of producing and distributing resources, but also the mechanism by which individual freedom will be protected and enhanced. The state, on the other hand, can never provide or allocate goods and services as efficiently as the market. Perhaps even more importantly, it is believed that state provision will restrict individual freedom by limiting individual choice and by imposing taxes to pay for the services provided. The key tenets of the neo-liberal strand of the New Right are thus freedom, choice, the individual, free markets and minimal state intervention (Joseph and Sumption 1979).

The second strand within the New Right has been referred to as neo-Conservative. This advocates a more interventionist role for the state in promoting traditional family values, morality, law and order, citizenship, duty, responsibility and community. A strong state is also thought to be necessary to provide the conditions within which the market can operate efficiently and effectively (Marsland, 1988: 4–9). Within this strand of the New Right is a concern that emphasising free market values could undermine important social norms and values. The essence of these two strands within the New Right are summarised by David Willetts in discussing the values of modern Conservatism:

> Conservatives appear to speak in two different languages. On the one hand they appeal to the individual, to initiative, enterprise and freedom. On the other hand there is the trust in community, deference, convention, authority. Many believe that these represent two fundamentally incompatible views of the world and that a set of free-market arrivistes have taken over the party of deference and authority. (Willetts, 1992: 181)

However, while tension exists between these two strands within the New Right, there is a shared belief that excessive state action, particularly in some forms of welfare provision, will be damaging for the individual, the family, the economy and society.

According to the New Right, the level of state welfare provided during and since the post-war period is excessive, inefficient and poorly directed and has resulted in a number of economic and social ills. The state has displaced the 'natural' sources of welfare provision, that is the market, families and philanthropy, and in doing so has also distorted the market's ability to operate optimally. The economic and social problems caused by such displacement could only be rectified, according to the New Right, by reducing state provision and reasserting the primacy of the natural, non-state sources of provision. It is not denied by the New Right that the state will need to provide some welfare services for those unable to make effective provision for themselves, or for those without family or community support. However, this would be a situation in which only a minority of people find themselves; the majority could and should be able to take care of their own needs or those of their families.

The cost of the NHS and state welfare provision have, according to the New Right, generally grown beyond the economy's ability to finance such expenditure. In the area of health care, where there is no price mechanism to control demand and medical advances lead to new and increased demands, the cost of provision is potentially infinite. As a related point, the New Right contends that the problem of funding the NHS has been exacerbated by inefficient use of limited resources by medical professionals intent on fuelling demand in their own self-interest. According to the New Right, any expansion of the welfare state, including the NHS, actually benefits the professionals employed within it, or those who are dependent on government contracts, more than the users of the service (see Chapter 7).

The absence of effective competition in the provision of health care not only creates the conditions for such inefficiency and pursuit of self-interest but also removes the incentives which, in a free market situation, ensure providers respond to the demands of their service users or consumers. The benefits derived from consumer sovereignty are negated by monopolistic state provision of health care (see Chapter 7). It is contended by the New Right that health care consumers have been denied any realistic freedom of choice in the area of health care since the inception of the NHS in 1948. Constraining individual freedom in this way is an unacceptable consequence of collective provision via the state and is of concern to the neo-liberal strand in particular, advocates of which place great emphasis on protecting and enhancing such freedom. State welfare provision, particularly that which is too generous or too accessible, has also made people less willing to take responsibility for their own or their family's welfare either through work, savings or insurance, thus becoming dependent on the state to meet all their needs. The New Right have therefore argued that the overextensive welfare state of the post-war period has created a number of problems, not the least of which are an over-burdened economy and a growing dependency culture.

According to the New Right, the solution to the economic, social and even political problems created by the welfare state is to reduce the level of state-provided services. The remaining lower level of state provision should be aimed at those who have no recourse to any other means of support. The majority of the population can and should provide for themselves via the market or rely on their family for support or philanthropy for assistance. Selective provision, however, means that some criteria must be devised for defining the target group and excluding those who are deemed ineligible. These criteria may take the form of a means-test, a special needs test, an age test, or some combination of these. Thus the New Right clearly advocate a residual role for the state as a welfare provider and increased roles for the private sector, the family, the voluntary sector and charities. This prescriptive element in the New Right perspective is aimed at reducing public expenditure, promoting economic growth, encouraging individual and family responsibility and enhancing individual freedom.

It has also been suggested by a number of writers from within this perspective that, had the state not intervened, the private sector, together with philanthropy, would have met the welfare needs of the majority in a more efficient and effective way than that in which welfare is currently provided (West, 1994; Green, 1994; Seldon, 1994). According to David Green (1994), apart from providing for the very poorest and protecting human freedom, there was no necessity for the state to interfere in what was an already improving non-state health care system, or to 'monopolise health provision' (21).

The popularity of the NHS, despite its problems, has made it politically difficult to implement any reforms which would radically interfere with the founding principles of comprehensive provision and universal access on the basis of citizenship. While it would seem difficult to privatise health care in any substantial way, there has been a concerted effort to return more peripheral services to the market and an attempt to 'marketise' the NHS. A fuller discussion of these issues can be found in Chapters 6 and 8.

Feminist Perspectives

Because of the different groupings and divisions within feminism, any attempt to offer one single feminist analysis of health care policy will prove overly simplistic. However, there are, as previously noted, certain themes within feminist analyses which draw these different groups together.

Feminists' attitudes towards health services have tended to be ambivalent. On the one hand, feminists have been highly critical of the way in which health care and welfare services generally have been provided. On the other hand, they recognise the benefits women have already gained from state provided health care and the potential of the welfare state to provide the means by which further benefits could be realised. Doyal (1985) argues that this ambivalence arises from the contradictory nature of health care services themselves: that women can gain much of value from the NHS, but also experience this state-provided service as oppressive.

Women are major users of health care services, primarily as the result of childbirth and longevity. Women are also major providers of health and social care, both within and outside the welfare state. Thus the creation of the NHS has provided women with access to health care, free at the point of use, as a citizenship right. The NHS has also provided paid employment for many women in a variety of occupations, as well as offering supportive services to women caring for relatives in their own home. However, despite the importance of health services in women's lives and the benefits women have derived from this provision, feminists remain highly critical of the way in which health care services are provided.

Feminist critiques of health care services are wide-ranging and the different strands within feminist analysis tend to focus on different aspects of provision. Liberal feminists have, for example, concerned themselves with promoting equality of opportunity and eradicating discrimination. Liberal feminists would therefore advocate equal access to all areas of medical training and all occupations within the health care system. They have campaigned for an end to discrimination in, amongst other things, recruitment and selection, wages and promotion. However liberal feminists tend to ignore the real differences between the lives of men and women. In particular they ignore the way in which gender roles mean that men's lives are primarily spent in the public sphere and women's in the private sphere. Advocating equality of opportunity within the public sphere, including the welfare state, will have little impact on women's lives, because it takes no account of their domestic role, a role which affects and constrains women's opportunities in the public sphere.

Socialist feminists, on the other hand, view women's domestic role and the unwaged labour associated with this as integral to any analysis of welfare provision and the position of women. According to socialist feminists, women's position is structured by the mutually supporting systems of patriarchy and capitalism. In this context of patriarchal capitalism, it is contended that women are assumed to live within a traditional family and be dependent on a male breadwinner. According to this strand of feminism, the unwaged role of women in social reproduction benefits capitalism by cutting the cost to capital of reproducing the next generation of wage labourers. Assumptions about women's dependency also mean that, if they are in paid work, they have a reduced earning capacity. Employers do not have to pay women as highly as men because women, unlike men, do not have to bear the full costs of providing for their own and their family's needs. Socialist feminists are therefore highly critical of welfare policy which supports the male breadwinner model of the family, a model which is functional for capitalism and perpetuates male power, but creates a subordinate position for women within both the domestic and public spheres.

Radical feminists contend that all women are oppressed by all men in a universal system of patriarchy. Women's oppression, according to this feminist approach, is rooted in biology and directly related to their sexual relationships with men in the domestic sphere. The welfare state is viewed as a means by which male domination can be maintained and perpetuated. The logic of this contention is that radical feminists typically argue for separate services for women, provided by women, such as well-woman clinics.

Feminists therefore contend that social policies, including health policies, have been based on a number of assumptions about women and their socially constructed roles. These assumptions have been neither questioned nor challenged by policy makers in the past and have therefore continued to shape and control the way in which women live their lives. For example, feminist research has demonstrated that the medical treatment and advice given to their women patients by some general practitioners has the effect of reinforcing the assumption that the primary, even natural, role for women is in the domestic sphere (Foster, 1991).

The system under which health care is provided is also said to be one in which doctors exercise patriarchal control over their female patients. Feminists have been highly critical of male-dominated mainstream health care and question whether women benefit as much as men from such a system. Feminists point out, for example, that doctors exercise this control in decisions concerning women's sexuality and their reproductive capacity (Ungerson, 1985: 149). Women suffering from female health problems such as pre-menstrual syndrome or menopausal symptoms have been dealt with unsympathetically by male general practitioners. Feminists have also been critical of the way in which mainstream medicine has tackled childbirth, for example, with the overuse of inductions and Caesarean sections, as well as other female issues such as hysterectomies and mastectomies. Doctors who expect their female patients to play a passive role, during consultations or medical treatments, are also an issue highlighted by feminists. Again the issue of childbirth provides a clear example of this expected passivity on the part of women. Women who have attempted to take a more active role in their own health care can be labelled as difficult patients by doctors. The way in which doctors view women's and men's symptoms in isolation from their social lives, when it may be a social problem causing the health problem, is another practice of which feminists are critical. For example, a woman complaining of stress-related symptoms can be prescribed tranquillisers when the health problem may stem from a social problem such as poor housing or male violence.

Feminists are therefore critical of the medical model of health care which dominates mainstream health care provision, both within the NHS and in many instances outside the state system. They advocate health care which takes a holistic view, promotes self-help and operates on a co-operative rather than a hierarchical basis: that is, health care which treats women as equals and enables them to participate in their own health care. This critique of mainstream medicine notwithstanding, feminists do not support arguments for cutting back the NHS. In fact feminists have been actively fighting threats to cut back resources allocated to health care. This defence largely reflects the serious effects for women of any cutbacks in this area. Women are both major users of the NHS and represent the majority of paid employees within the service. Additionally, reductions in NHS provision can further increase the level of unpaid caring work women undertake at home. Feminists therefore advocate changing the way in which health care is provided rather than reducing the level of provision: the latter would simply further disadvantage women.

Marxist Perspectives

Within Marxism there are, as within other perspectives, a number of different schools of thought providing a variety of analyses of the welfare state and social policies. However, Marxists generally adhere to the view that the stated aims of welfare provision will never be achieved within the context of a capitalist system.

Marxist writers contend that it is neither possible, nor was it the intention of the social democratic welfare state, to achieve greater equality through redistributive social policies. According to Marxists, the development of the welfare state was not primarily an attempt to pursue greater equality by, for example, ameliorating poverty, ill-health or ignorance within the working class. Rather the welfare state developed in response to the changing needs of a dynamic capitalist system; needs which were not being met by the market alone. Although Marxists do not deny that the working class have derived some benefits from the provision of welfare services, this is seen to be of only marginal significance in a service designed to support the market system of exchange and capital accumulation. It has been argued, for example, that the priorities of the NHS have always reflected the interests of capital rather than the real needs of patients (Doyal, 1979: 185–6).

Until relatively recently, Marxist writers failed to analyse the welfare state in any detail. Until about the 1970s, welfare provision was treated by Marxists as either a concession made by capital in times of labour unrest or as a minor victory won by the working class. However, in the early 1970s, the debate between Miliband and Poulantzas (see Blackburn, 1972) concerning the role and degree of autonomy of the state, together with the writing of O'Connor (1973) and Gough (1979), led to the development of a coherent Marxist analysis of the welfare state.

For many contemporary Marxist writers the emergence of a welfare state reflects the successful use of the state by capitalists to ensure the conditions necessary for capital accumulation. That is, capitalists have used the state to help them tackle problems thrown up by the capitalist system itself, problems which market systems were failing to address adequately. These problems included, for example, the ill-health and low level of education amongst the working class, when what was needed by capitalism was a healthy workforce with a higher level of skills.

The welfare state, according to Marxists, also assists capital by helping to maintain social harmony and the legitimacy of the capitalist system. The operation of free market forces can produce consequences which could lead to discontent: consequences such as high levels of unemployment, poverty in old age, homelessness, ill-health and a lack of affordable health care services. With provision being made for such contingencies in the form of income mainte-nance, pensions, housing and a universally accessible health care system, Marxists contend that discontent is subdued and stable conditions for capital accumulation can be secured. Initially, there-fore, many Marxist writers analysed the welfare state in terms of the functions it provided for a capitalist system. However, from about the 1970s, the functional role of a welfare state was challenged and criticised by a number of contemporary Marxists.

Much of the neo-Marxist analysis of the welfare state is concerned with the dysfunctional role of state welfare provision in capitalist societies (see, for example, O'Connor, 1973; Gough, 1979). Although differences exist between neo-Marxists, they argue in essence that ultimately the growth of state welfare provision will threaten capit-alism, the very system which the welfare state was developed to protect. The detailed steps in this 'crisis' strand of neo-Marxist analysis are comprehensively presented in O'Connor's (1973) writ-ing; the main themes of his analysis are briefly outlined here. O'Connor argues that there are two main categories of public exp-enditure, which he labels as social capital and social expenses. Social capital refers to investment by the state in two main areas, physical capital which includes expenditure on, for example, roads and rail-ways, and human capital which includes expenditure on, for exam-ple, education and health. Both areas of social capital expenditure are part of what O'Connor refers to as the state's accumulation function.

Social expenses may not directly benefit capitalism in the way that social capital does, but indirectly state expenditure in this area also benefits capital accumulation by maintaining stable social conditions. State expenditure on, for example, retirement pensions, unemploy-ment benefit or health care help to mitigate some of the most unacceptable problems existing in society. These problems often result from the operation of markets, as with poverty created by unemployment or low wages, but the market alone does not provide any socially acceptable solutions. While social expenses may be a drain on profitability in the short term, in that revenue is derived from taxes, in the longer term such expenditure supports capitalism by maintaining the legitimacy and thus stability of the system. O'Connor refers to this second function of the state as its 'legitimation function'.

Public expenditure on health care could be viewed as social capital, in that it helps to maintain a healthy workforce needed by capitalism, or as social expenses, in that it provides health care for everyone and thus helps legitimise the capitalist system. In either case capitalism benefits from the state provision of health care. As Navarro (1976) states:

> there is no clear-cut dichotomy between the social needs of capital and the social demands of labour. Any given policy can serve both. Indeed, social policies that serve the interests of the working class can be subsequently adapted to benefit the interests of the dominant class. (220–1)

Continuing demand from the labour movement for increased expenditure on health and other social services results in responses from both capitalists and the state: 'It is important to stress that these responses always take place within the context of the primary function of the state, which is to ensure the process of capital accumulation' (Navarro, 1978: 85).

However, problems arise when the level of expenditure on welfare provision continues to grow, necessitating concomitant increases in taxation to fund expanded state provision. However, unlike the New Right, Marxists do not believe it will be possible to reduce levels of public expenditure in order to protect profitability without undermining the other important function of the state, which is to maintain the legitimacy of the capitalist system. Once the state significantly reduces expenditure on welfare provision, the legitimacy of capitalism can no longer be assured. If the legitimacy of the system is challenged or threatened, the system may become unstable, a condition which is not conducive to profit accumulation. It is therefore argued by neo-Marxist writers that the welfare state occupies a contradictory position (Gough, 1979), in that it is both functional and dysfunctional for capitalism. The welfare state which developed to solve the problems inherent in capitalist systems has, according to Marxists, sown the seeds of its own destruction (Mishra, 1984).

Welfare Pluralist Perspective

The concept of welfare pluralism, increasingly referred to as the mixed economy of welfare, has grown in importance in debates about social policy from the late 1970s. The first time that the term 'welfare pluralism' was used was probably in 1978 with the publication of the Wolfenden Report, but the first major discussion of welfare pluralism was provided by Gladstone (1979). It is difficult to provide an accurate definition of welfare pluralism as a number of arguments and explanations have been offered under this label. However the definition offered by Hatch and Mocroft seems to provide a useful starting point:

> In one sense welfare pluralism can be used to convey the fact that social and health care may be obtained from four different sectors – the statutory, the voluntary, the commercial and the informal. More prescriptively welfare pluralism implies a less dominant role for the state, seeing it as not the only possible instrument for the collective provision of welfare services. As far as local authorities are concerned, this suggests policies which recognise and seek to reinforce other sources of care rather than relying on statutory action in isolation from them. (Hatch and Mocroft, 1983: 2)

Many leading proponents of welfare pluralism emphasise the need to maximise voluntary and community based welfare provision as alternatives to state provision (Hadley and Hatch, 1981; Hatch and Mocroft, 1983). The commercial sector is also believed to have a role, albeit a more limited one, to play in the provision of welfare. However commercial provision must be subject to safeguards to maintain quality and cannot be allowed to affect other sources of service provision detrimentally (Hadley and Hatch, 1981).

Welfare pluralists are not so much critical of the principle of collective provision, rather the form in which collective provision has been made (Hadley and Hatch, 1981: 3). Welfare pluralists question the assumption that the state should occupy a central role in the provision of welfare services. This assumption is questioned because state welfare provision, despite increased expenditure and extended social services, has failed to achieve its original goals, such as improved health care provision for everyone and a reduction in inequalities. These authors are also critical of the way in which the statutory sector behaves as though it is the only provider of services, a situation which they claim does not reflect reality. According to Hadley and Hatch (1981), therefore, the achievements of social services do not seem to justify the level of public funding received by these services.

Proponents of welfare pluralism are concerned to differentiate their views from those of the New Right. The fact that welfare pluralists advocate a reduced role for the state in the provision of welfare services, as do proponents of the New Right, does not mean that these two perspectives are interchangeable. Welfare pluralists propose a way forward which they claim differentiates their mixed economy approach from both the political right and the left. Rather than idealistically promoting market provision, or continuing to support state provision as a virtual monopoly despite its shortcomings, welfare pluralists advocate both pluralistic and decentralised welfare services.

In pursuing a mixed economy of welfare, welfare pluralists advocate expansion of the services provided by the voluntary and informal sectors. However, while welfare pluralists are concerned about further expansion of the commercial sector, this sector, too, is seen to have a role to play in providing welfare services. Most welfare pluralists accept that the state will continue to have a significant role, although not as a major service provider. The role prescribed for the state, from this perspective, is strategic and regulatory. The state is viewed as the agency with the ability to facilitate and regulate the development of the roles of alternative providers and to ensure that priorities and standards of service provision are maintained.

Welfare pluralism has been inseparably linked to policies of community care and thus the expansion of the social care market. Social services departments, rather than the NHS, have been the areas of the welfare state where welfare pluralist perspectives have been most influential. However the interdependence of health and social care, particularly with the implementation of community care policies, means that the way in which social care services are provided has potentially significant effects on the NHS. The level of social care can affect the NHS in terms of discharge rates, admissions, readmissions, pressure on acute beds and waiting list targets, to highlight just some areas in the secondary health care sector alone (Wistow *et al.*, 1994).

Anti-Racist Perspectives

Explanations of continuing racial inequalities have not been integrated into mainstream social policy debates to the extent that explanations of class and subsequently gender inequalities have been. Evidence concerning the disadvantaged position of Britain's non-white population, as both employees and service users, has come from many areas of the welfare state, however.

The overrepresentation of black and Asian workers within the lower status, lower paid sections of the labour force, both inside and outside the welfare state, has been well documented (see Skellington, 1992). This is a situation which is reflected within the NHS itself, where black and Asian workers are performing less skilled tasks and are disproportionately found in the less prestigious areas of medicine (Kushnik, 1988). Statistics specifically concerning the health of black and Asian communities are not officially recorded. However individual experiences of racism within the NHS have been recorded in various accounts and include, amongst others, discriminatory experiences in clinical consultations, nursing care and in general practice (Donovan, 1986).

The explanations for this continuing disadvantage, from within a broadly anti-racist perspective, take a variety of forms. Radical explanations claim that not only is racism inherent in British society but this racism is intentionally perpetuated by the state. Racist ideologies, according to this view, inform both policy and practice and because racism, insofar as it maintains divisions between the white and non-white population, is functional for capitalism there is no concerted attempt to tackle it.

Racism, it is contended, can benefit capitalist systems in a number of ways, one important and obvious example being the additional recruits racism provides for capitalism's reserve army of labour. The existence of racism has meant, moreover, that ethnic minority groups can be used as scapegoats and blamed for a range of problems, from increasing unemployment to the inadequacy of welfare services. The benefit to capitalism is that criticism is diverted from the system. Without racism, criticism which would have been directed at the market system of allocation or, alternatively, at central government policies which limit the resources going into the welfare state, is redirected to ethnic minority groups who are believed to 'abuse' welfare services.

The state has effectively reinforced the view that the presence of non-white groups in the population is a problem. For example, the state has implemented immigration legislation which has had the effect, and according to radical anti-racists the intention, of limiting the numbers of non-white immigrants entering Britain (see CCCS, 1982). Such legislation, implemented by successive governments, is said to legitimise the belief that the presence of ethnic minorities in Britain is a problem: otherwise why should Britain try to limit the numbers of non-white people entering the country?

The 'problematic' presence of ethnic minority groups has taken a particularly acute form in relation to the welfare state. Any recent non-white immigrants, and by association all of Britain's ethnic minority population, have become depicted as people who overutilise and thus reduce the scarce resources of the welfare state, whose entitlement to welfare services is at best questionable and whose use of welfare services needs to be vigilantly policed in order to prevent them abusing the system.

While radical perspectives focus on a fairly narrow range of issues in their explanations of racial disadvantage and inequalities, there are alternative explanations from within this anti-racist perspective which incorporate a broader range of factors. The issues raised and explanations offered by radical commentators are important, but in limiting their analysis to issues which have a high profile, such as immigration controls and law and order policy, radical commentators fail to examine the detailed and complex means by which racial disadvantage is often perpetuated by many social institutions, including those of the welfare state. It has been argued that 'there can be two levels at which racism operates: at the level of policies, rules or their interpretation, and at another level in the refusal to acknowledge racism and/or do something about it' (Ben-Tovim *et al.*, 1986: 22). In addition to the above, racial disadvantage and inequality can be perpetuated either intentionally, by direct discrimination, or unintentionally, through indirect discrimination. Examples of all of these processes can be found within the welfare state itself.

One of the founding principles of the welfare state and thus the NHS was universalism. As a guiding principle, universalism supports the view that everyone should be treated equally, irrespective of class, colour or creed, that a 'colour-blind' approach to welfare provision should be adopted. This approach, however, has had the, albeit unintended, effect of reinforcing existing inequalities. Adopting a universalist approach leads to a failure to recognise and act upon the particular and specific needs of ethnic minority groups (see Chapter 7). Within the NHS this could lead to a failure to respond to certain dietary needs, the failure to provide interpreters or to acknowledge any cultural differences, the result of which will be that members of ethnic minority groups are disadvantaged, although this may never have been the intention.

If, in addition to the failure to respond to the specific needs of ethnic minorities, welfare professionals are also influenced by negative stereotypes of ethnic minorities and their cultures, this could influence policies and the way in which they are interpreted and implemented by welfare professionals. A 'colour-blind' approach within policies, or negative stereotypical views of ethnic minorities, can lead to a situation where there is institutional resistance to complaints of racial discrimination and harassment. This resistance may take the form of failing to implement effective mechanisms for monitoring and dealing with such complaints or of blaming the victim rather than the perpetrator.

In addition to being disadvantaged as consumers of welfare services, ethnic minorities as welfare producers also occupy a disadvantaged position. This disadvantage may result from direct discrimination in terms of personnel recruitment, selection and appointment, or from indirect discrimination arising from pursuing traditional policies and practices (see Chapter 7) . For example, the practice of requiring a personal recommendation from a senior consultant, before appointment to the staff of a hospital, could produce discriminatory outcomes for members of ethnic minority groups who do not have the necessary network of contacts.

From within this strand of anti-racism, therefore, the continuation of racial disadvantage is explained by the interaction of a broader and more complex range of factors than those outlined by radical anti-racists. The central state is again implicated in the failure to eradicate racial inequalities, not as radical anti-racists claim, by intent, but rather by default. The central state appears to have devolved responsibility for implementing a number of anti-racist measures to the local state and the discretion of professionals within the public sector. In doing so the central state appears to have attempted to distance itself from the issues around racial divisions and inequalities and has failed to provide the central lead necessary if anti-racist initiatives are to be effective in eliminating discrimination and disadvantage.

Conclusion

Having briefly examined a number of perspectives which have been used to analyse health policy and practice, it is clear that each one offers a distinctive approach to analysis, a specific focus of debate and related to this, a prescription for the future of health care. Each perspective contends that there are certain problems with the way in which health care is currently structured and provided and changes are proposed which address and, it is hoped, rectify these. The perspectives will be revisited and applied to particular health care issues in the following chapters, where the rather stark theoretical outlines provided in this chapter will be developed by the addition of examples and discussion.

Bibliography

Abel-Smith, B. and Townsend, P. (1965) *The Poor and the Poorest: a new analysis of the Ministry of Labour's family expenditure surveys of 1953–54 and 1960*, London: Bell.

Ben-Tovim, G., Gabriel, J., Law, I. and Stredder, K. (1986) *The Local Politics of Race*, London: Macmillan.

Beveridge, W. H. (1942) *Social Insurance and Allied Services*, Cmd 6404, London: HMSO.

Black, Sir Douglas (1982) *Inequalities in Health: The Black Report*, Harmondsworth: Penguin.

Blackburn, R. (ed.) (1972) *Ideology in Social Science*, London: Fontana.

Bryson, L. (1992) *Welfare and the State*, Basingstoke: Macmillan.

CCCS (Centre for Contemporary Cultural Studies) (1982) *The Empire Strikes Back, Race and Racism in 70's Britain*, London: Hutchinson University Library.

Crosland, C. A. R. (1956) *The Future of Socialism*, London: Cape.

Donovan, J. (1986) *We Don't Buy Sickness, It Just Comes: Health Illness and Health Care in the Lives of Black People in London*, Aldershot: Gower.

Doyal, L. (1979) *The Political Economy of Health*, London: Pluto Press.

Doyal, L. (1985) 'Women and the Crisis in the National Health Service', in C. Ungerson (ed.), *Women and Social Policy*, Basingstoke: Macmillan.

Foster, P. (1991) 'Well Women Clinics: A Serious Challenge to Mainstream Health Care', in M. Maclean and D. Groves (eds), *Women's Issues in Social Policy*, London: Routledge.

George, V. and Wilding, P. (1994) *Welfare and Ideology*, Hemel Hempstead: Harvester Wheatsheaf.

Gladstone, F. J. (1979) *Voluntary Action in a Changing World*, London: Bedford: Square Press.

Glennerster, H. (1992) *Paying for Welfare: The 1990s*, Hemel Hempstead: Harvester Wheatsheaf.

Gough, I. (1979) *Political Economy of the Welfare State*, Basingstoke: Macmillan.

Green, D. G. (1988) *Everyone a Private Patient*, London: Institute of Economic Affairs.

Green, D. G. (1994) 'Medical Care Before the NHS', *Economic Affairs*, vol. 14, no. 5, pp. 21–4.

Hadley, R. and Hatch, S. (1981) *Social Welfare and the Failure of the State: Centralised Social Services and Participatory Alternatives*, London: Allen & Unwin.

Hatch, S. and Mocroft, L. (1983) *Components of Welfare: voluntary organisations, social services and politics in two local authorities*, London: Bedford Square, Press/NCVO.

Hill, M. and Bramley, G. (1986) *Analysing Social Policy*, London: Basil Blackwell.

HMSO (1944) *A National Health Service*, February, Cmd 6502 White Paper, London: HMSO.

Joseph, K. and Sumption, J. (1979) *Equality*, London: John Murray.

Kushnick, L. (1988) 'Racism, the National Health Service and the Health of Black People', *International Journal of Health Services*, vol. 18, no. 3.

Marshall, T. H. (1975) *Social Policy*, 4th edn, London: Hutchinson University Library.

Marsland, D. (1988) 'The Welfare State as a Producer Monopoly', *Salisbury Review*, no. 6.

Miliband, R. (1973) 'Reply to Nicos Poulantzas', in R. Blackburn (ed.), *Ideology in Social Science*, London: Fontana/Collins.

Mishra, R. (1984) *The Welfare State in Crisis: Social Thought and Social Change*, Brighton: Wheatsheaf

Navarro, V. (1976) *Medicine Under Capitalism*, London: Croom Helm.

Navarro, V. (1978) *Class Struggle, the State and Medicine*, London: Martin Robertson.

O'Connor, J. (1973) *The Fiscal Crisis of the State*, London: St James Press.

Seldon, A. (1994) 'Saving for Life-time Risks', *Economic Affairs*, vol. 14, no. 5.

Skellington, R. (1992) *Race in Britain Today*, London: Sage and Open University Press.

Titmuss R. M. (1963) *Essays on the Welfare State*, 2nd edn, London: Unwin University Books.

Titmuss R. M. (1970) *The Gift Relationship*, Bungay, Suffolk: George Allen & Unwin.

Titmuss, R. M. (1976) *Commitment to Welfare*, 2nd edn, Bungay, Suffolk: George Allen & Unwin.

Ungerson, C. (1985) 'Introduction to Women and the Crisis in the National Health Service', in C. Ungerson (ed.), *Women and Social Policy*, Basingstoke: Macmillan.

West, E. G. (1994) 'Education Without the State', *Economic Affairs*, vol. 14, no. 5.

Willetts, D. (1992) *Modern Conservatism*, London:Penguin Books.

Williams, F. (1989) *Social Policy: A Critical Introduction*, Cambridge: Polity.

Wilson, E. (1977) *Women and the Welfare State*, London: Tavistock.

Wistow, G., Knapp, M., Hardy, B. and Allen, C. (1994) *Social Care in a Mixed Economy*, Buckingham: Open University Press.

Wolfenden, Lord (1978) *The Future of Voluntary Organisations*, Report of the Committee on the Future of Voluntary Organisations, London: Croom Helm.

2

Policy Processes

Nancy North

Whenever a policy is announced, whether it be a different approach to economic affairs, enabling schools to 'opt out' or creating an internal market in health care, there is usually a great deal of media and academic speculation on its probable outcomes and rather less concern about how and why the policy emerged. This chapter attempts to redress the balance by outlining a range of theories which have offered explanations about the process of making policy. It will end by raising some key issues which will be revisited in subsequent chapters.

There is little point in talking about the processes of policy making without first trying to clarify what 'policy' is, but unfortunately this is a far from easy task. Policies could be said to be both a statement of the current view of an issue and an attempt to standardise future actions or responses in relation to that issue. So far so good, but policies come in different guises and whilst it may be possible to identify a core to policy, its scope may be somewhat indeterminable. In addition White Papers, such as *Working for Patients* (Department of Health, 1989), may offer conceptual terra firma in that they are proposed policies which governments may later enshrine in law, but other policies materialise less obviously. Jacob (1991) points out the importance of binding circulars issued by health ministers: if health authorities choose to ignore these the Secretary of State has the right to intervene. Within the NHS, guidance issued by the National Health Service Management Executive (NHSME), while not having the force of law or formal sanction, nevertheless carries a great deal of influence. It is unlikely that either executive or non-executive members of health authorities would wish to be seen as rebels.

23

Policy making is not the prerogative of central government alone. Those who have migrated between jobs in the NHS will be aware that policies initiated at the local level can result in very different working environments. Given the slippery nature of the concept, perhaps the most appropriate description is that of a former mandarin of the Civil Service who suggested that policy was like an elephant, recognisable when seen but not easily defined (cited in Ham and Hill, 1993).

Difficulties also arise when the process of policy making is examined. The details of government policies are left to civil servants to determine and execute. In the case of the NHS – a state institution – they do so in part by issuing documents which guide or instruct the various elements within the service and through discussions with senior managers and elected members at district and, until 1996, regional health authority levels. The distinction between informing about and participating in policy making is not always clear. Furthermore managers and the District Health Authorities (DHAs) to whom they are responsible may reinterpret, embellish or make additions to government policies, a process which in theory has been encouraged by the devolution of decision making in the NHS. This may result in different forms of provision, although the central government could stipulate minimum levels or standards. For example, when DHAs were enabled, by the NHS and Community Care Act 1990, to change the pattern of services in their catchment area, a small number decided to end provision for male sterilisations within the NHS. Presumably not wishing to encourage unplanned fatherhood, the government acted quickly to reinstate the service and reinforced the need for acceptable levels of family planning. Decisions about who provides the service (GPs and/or specialist NHS or voluntary family planning centres) and the level of provision remain a matter of local health purchaser discretion.

As well as the managers and the elected members of an authority, there is another group through which policies in health care are filtered – these are the professionals working within the health service. The concept of clinical autonomy has permitted the medical profession in particular a great deal of discretionary power (see Chapters 3 and 8). In the past, governments both recognised and endorsed this. Other than acknowledging the significance of medical decision making and imploring the profession to engage more in management, they tended to leave the volatile issue of clinical autonomy alone.

However every clinical decision to treat a patient has resource implications. As an adjunct of the need to control health care expenditure, a preoccupation of many industrialised states which will be discussed in the Chapter 8, concern about the clinical effectiveness of treatments has also grown. The resulting emphasis on the dissemination of research on cost-effectiveness and on clinical audit is likely to encourage the use of treatment protocols and local policies on service development. In Chapters 5 and 6 these issues are discussed further.

The discussion so far has given some idea of the difficulties of conceptualising policy making as something which is produced centrally and carried out unequivocally. Quite apart from the reinterpretation of policy through the implementation process, the business of running the modern state makes it impossible for central government to determine or oversee the local interpretation of policies. Despite this, a central government can establish conditions which exert considerable influence over the way local policies develop. The above description of an essentially top-down, albeit multi-layered, process conveys neither an impression of events leading up to the announcement of a policy nor the confusion, pragmatism and purposeful negotiations which may continue afterwards. The image of considered and judicious policy emerging effortlessly from government is as naive as the child's perception of babies arriving with the stork. The gestation of the NHS Bill, in 1946, was a more tortured process than that, but even this phase of policy making did not compare with Bevan's subsequent negotiations with the medical profession (Eckstein, 1960; Willcocks, 1967; Klein, 1989) which will be discussed further in Chapters 3 and 5. Neither does relative tranquillity in the initial stages of policy development signify contented acquiescence; governments may decide not to consult and may exclude traditional partners from the policy making process, let alone the never-rans.

Clearly power in one form or another is central to any explanation of policy making, whether it is demonstrated in the countervailing pressures a government brings to bear to confine the creativity of DHAs within acceptable limits, or in the previously impregnable authority of the medical profession, wielded with great effect in committees at all levels of the NHS. Power and its relationships will be elaborated in the next section, but before this important topic is addressed some qualification of the discussion thus far is advisable. By focusing on key events in the history of the NHS this discussion has tended to theorise policy making, like the creation of the universe, as a 'big-bang' affair: in other words, as a process which brings about transcendent and radical change. With a few esoteric exceptions, such as the application of new genetic technologies, modern policy making rarely has the advantage of an empty universe and must address the outcomes of past policies. This is a task which inevitably limits the potential for, or speed of, change. Additionally radical change requires varying proportions of political courage, public support (or its manipulation) and financial resources. Governments may be unwilling to take such risks.

The remainder of this chapter will outline a series of explanatory theories about policy making which will develop the discussion above. They will provide different perspectives on the policy-making process, but, in offering a simplified view of reality, no one theory is perfect. Their value lies in the fact that they help to establish important questions about the nature of policy making in the health service rather than offering unassailable explanations. Before diving head-long into the theories it is necessary to discuss a concept which is fundamental to all policy-making power.

Power

One's view about whether the distribution of power in society is pluralistic (widely dispersed), elitist (concentrated) or somewhere in between rather depends upon how power is recognised. Power, or the ability to influence another's actions, is most easily identified, whether in the guise of military threat, an influential piece of lobbying or a decision taken by a legitimate authority, when the process is visible. A concentration upon tangible displays of power led some theorists to adopt an inadequate view of political processes. The significance of covert power and agenda setting – non-decisions resulting in the marginalisation of issues – was identified by Bachrach and Baratz (1970). Elaborating on the work of an earlier author (Schattschneider), Bachrach and Baratz recognised the significance of dominant values and beliefs in excluding minority interests from decision making processes. This is not merely a question of not being heard; some issues may not be articulated because of the fear of retribution. For example, staff may want to address what they perceive as inadequate funding for a service but are reluctant to point this out to decision-making bodies. Another way of controlling decision making is to co-opt the potential opposition. Consumer groups may be invited to participate in service planning meetings to head off vociferous objections to policy, though once incorporated in the process they may find their attempts frustrated by regulations and the skilful manoeuvrings of other members. Power is also personal: an opponent who is articulate, charismatic and has status can readily undermine a legitimate claim to be heard.

The contribution of Bachrach and Baratz moves the analysis of power on, from the evaluation of observable behaviour to a consideration of conflicting issues which, though articulated, remain outside the decision-making agenda. However, Lukes (1974) extends the idea of covert power further, arguing that potential issues are excluded from political debate because dominant interests succeed in neutralising them through the manipulation of public consciousness. Marginalised groups, whose interests otherwise would be promoted through the politicisation of key issues, thus remain oblivious to them. The manipulation of public consciousness is achieved through the dominance of ideology. Society's faith in the biomedical model of health care, espoused and promoted by the medical profession, secured a critical role in health policy making for the latter in the creation of the NHS and subsequently. From this perspective the fates of ideology and profession are entwined; the legitimacy of the medical profession as altruistic decision makers was sustained until criticisms of both the profession and the health care it promoted undermined the symbiotic relationship between state and profession. Views of health care such as those advanced by McKeown (1980) constituted an 'alternative consciousness' to the dominant medical model. This more critical approach to medicine's claims has been reconfigured in the growing interest in evidence based medicine, a concept which has acquired increasing currency in policy making. Debates about health care provision relating to more or less health promotion, screening and community care or transplants are framed within broader orthodoxies concerned with efficiency and effectiveness (see Chapter 6). 'Low-tech' programmes have to establish their worth, as do heart transplant and infertility programmes. Just as the power of the medical model is increasingly circumscribed by considerations of its efficacy – its ability to deliver predetermined outcomes in health – so too is the power of the medical profession.

This discussion has tried to relate theories of power to issues within health care, but it is important to recognise that the work of Bachrach and Baratz and of Lukes applies to debates about who controls the state, as well as who influences health policy in the UK or within the local DHAs. This will become clearer as these theories are outlined later in this chapter, but we begin with a group of theories which rather neglect the notion of power. They are included, not only because they provide a basis for comparison with other theories, but because organisations within both the public and private sector try to be and seem rational. Adopting an apparently rational process is assumed to be the means of securing the elusive goal of rationality.

Rational and Quasi-rational Theories of Decision Making

In the *Republic*, an ancient treatise on government, Plato suggested that only a highly educated (and male) elite, skilled in philosophic discourse, would possess the necessary knowledge and skills to rule. This association between policy making, the desirability of rational process and elite rather than democratic decision making lingers on in government and public administration, if not as a qualification for government then as a symbolic demonstration of fitness to govern.

At the risk of stating the obvious, theories of rational decision making assume that individuals are intrinsically rational. The criteria for rationality are minimal: 'consistency among goals and objectives . . . consistency in the application of principles in order to select the optimal alternative' (Allison, 1971: 29). The elusive but desirable goal of rationality is confirmed by way of the process of decision making. Theories of rational decision making confidently require that decision makers identify a problem or goal, consider the possible solutions, estimate the consequences of each course of action and select the strategy that best fits the policy goal. According to Minogue (1983), managerialism has attached great importance to rational decision making processes, even to the degree that it employs mechanisms such as cost–benefit analysis to help to rationalise the process of choosing between options. This is a false hope: the values of those constructing or interpreting such formula-based aids inevitably pervade the outcomes.

Rational theories of decision making are flawed because they demand too much of the decision makers and the state of knowledge. Human cognition and the ability to process information logically are limited and frequently unable to deal with the quantities of information which confronts policy makers. Like the top-down model of policy making and implementation, rational theories have been criticised for oversimplifying a complex and iterative process. However, the most fundamental criticism of all is the underlying assumption that rational thought is value-free and that decisions are thus logical rather than political. The response of hopeful pragmatists who support the notion of rationality is to suggest that the process of analysis will dissolve conflicts of interest. This is tantamount to saying that logical discussion will result in all seeing reason in the end, an assumption which conveniently ignores the fact that the solution is likely to reflect the view of those who have the most influence. Critics such as Lindblom (1959) also argue that this is an unrealistic view of what is essentially a political process. His views find empirical support in studies of the NHS. Hunter, commenting on the difficulties of the process of NHS planning in the 1970s, observed that there were 'multiple perceptions of rationality' (1980: 40).

Though some would argue that the descriptive power of the rational model is limited, its significance lies in its attribution as both an ideal type – a handy benchmark for researchers – or as a normative model. In other words, organisations and individuals strive to approximate rational decision making. The centralised NHS planning cycles of the 1970s, a managerial approximation of rationalism, have been abandoned, but in a series of publications the NHSME has enjoined DHA purchasers to follow seemingly rational procedures (see, for example, NHSME, 1991a, 1991b).

Incrementalism

Lindblom, one of the greatest scourges of the rational model, argued that policy making, far from being a confidently precise and rational process unsullied by everyday politics, was more pragmatic, uncertain and value-ridden. He suggested that policy makers focused on problem resolution rather than more ambitious goals. Having considered a limited number of well-tested options, they select a course of action which changes policy only marginally. Lindblom (1959) characterised this process of policy making as 'muddling through'. There is evidence that the NHS review which preceded the White Paper, *Working for Patients* (Department of Health, 1989), began by considering more radical alternatives for the NHS. Proposals to change to an insurance-based scheme were tabled, though the small ministerial team eventually settled on the option to create an internal market (Butler,1992). However, some would argue that this action was quite radical enough.

In response to critics who suggested that muddling through resulted in conservatism and could not cope with unusual crises, Lindblom (1979) reworked his theory. He discriminated between incremental analysis (shaping a policy) and incremental politics (the political will to endorse policy). He also argued that the dissemination of analytic work amongst various interested groups would permit complex problems to be resolved. Lindblom's concept of partisan mutual *adjustment* (PMA), describes a process whereby policies emerge in a system of decentralised decision making in which interested parties adjust their position in order to offset opposition and secure some measure of success. Accordingly agreements are hammered out by a process of rational debate, a nevertheless more impassioned process than the logical discussions characterising the rational models. Thus Lindblom claimed that his approach was capable of producing both rational and radical results.

The emphasis in Lindblom's 'muddling through' model on the political nature of decision making, distinguishes it from other rational decision making models. Lindblom's theory also stresses the incremental character of policy making. Both Ham (1992: 127) and Harrison (1988: 46) identify an incremental approach to policy making within the NHS, although Harrison rejects the concept of partisan mutual adjustment as an appropriate description of the key relationships between managers and the medical profession. The unspoken assumption in Lindblom's model is that PMA reflects a political process which is essentially pluralist: namely, that power in society is widely dispersed and interested groups have ease of access to the process of policy making. This has never been the case in the NHS and, even as a conceptualisation of democracy, unqualified pluralism has long since been discredited, as Lindblom recognised (Lindblom and Woodhouse, 1993). Patently, any discussion of policy making has to address rigorously the notion of power, who holds it, how it is exercised, why it is exercised and the consequences of its use.

Policies by Default: Routines in Decision Making

Allison's Bureaucratic or Organisational Process model (BPM) suggests that within organisations the presence of routines or standard operating procedures (SOPs), which are applied to specific issues, have a strong influence over policy. In other words organisational culture, structure and bureaucracy predetermine policy outputs. Arguably the origins of routines lie in past quasi-rational processes which select the best available solutions and, over time, repertoires of preferred actions are established. They are, in other words, the ossified products of past debates, endowing policy implementation with conservatism. The government's role is limited. According to Allison, government actors can interfere with organisations, but not control their behaviour. However, he recognised that arm's-length control could be exercised by specifying evaluative criteria and operating a system of 'rewards and punishments' (Allison, 1971: 86).

There are clear similarities between the above strategy and the measures introduced to regulate performance in the NHS (see Chapter 5), the results of which can only increase control of the central government over the implementation of critical aspects of policy (Klein, 1989; Paton, 1993). Although Allison and Lindblom both identify the political nature of policy making, their models are premised on very specific conceptualisations of power. The focus of Allison's study was on decision making within government during a crisis in state security (the Cuban missile crisis). Under these circumstances one would not expect lengthy debate or wide consultation outside specific government departments. Issues about the dissemination of power within the state therefore do not apply. Lindblom, on the other hand, does give the sense of widely dispersed decision making in policy processes, although in later publications he conceded that power was more likely to be concentrated within elite groups. Debates about the distribution of power within the state (macro-level theories) are important to an understanding of policy making and will now be investigated.

Power within the State

Pluralism, which conceives of power as disseminated within society, has focused on the observable activity of pressure groups within a political process which is essentially competitive. Dunleavy describes the pluralist view of power as widely distributed amongst interest groups who play a vital role in correcting the imbalances of power created by majority rule, since voluble opposition from a minority interest may result in some adjustment to policies. Debate, leading to consensus, is fundamental to the policy process, the 'power' of argument rather than structural economic or political power being influential. The state, whose boundaries are hard to establish but which encompasses government, state bureaucracies (such as the NHS), the judiciary, police and military, has a mediatory role which is deemed to be neutral yet responsive (Dunleavy, 1981, 1988).

Pluralism's somewhat anodyne view of the democratic state has been criticised, but the critics themselves have been castigated for attacking a model of pluralism which was but a caricature of the theory (Smith, 1990). Despite a spirited defence in which the divisions between pluralism and neo-pluralism become increasingly equivocal, there remain many weaknesses with pluralism's case. The assumption that access to government is reasonably open and that such access denotes legitimacy, is flawed. Smith suggests that, although pluralists recognise the unequal distribution of power, they fail to recognise the significance of ideological hegemony, which enables dominant interests to sustain a presence in policy making. Moreover the concentration on the responsiveness of the state to pressure groups disregards the possibility of the state as initiator of policy – a perspective which seems to be contradicted by more recent events in the UK. The 1970s neo-liberalist, anti-statist critiques, which viewed pluralism as the engine of increasingly ungovernable democracies, have been realised in Thatcherism's preference for selective restriction of interest group access to central government, as was evident in discussions leading to the 1990 NHS reforms.

Some theories have attempted to accommodate the dissonance between the pluralist view of events with accounts which identify the unequal access of groups to policy making (Hirst, 1987) and the existence of some relatively closed relationships between interest groups and government. Neo-pluralism recognises that the growth in the state's responsibilities has forced governments to devolve important policy decisions to other elements of the state such as locally elected authorities or authorised agencies and professional groups working within them. Two broad views exist. Firstly, professionals are seen as being committed to the public interest and can therefore be relied upon to substitute for political control. Further-more the extension of the state under welfare professionals and the resulting fragmentation of centres of power mitigate against the development of controlling elites (Dunleavy, 1988). However critiques of professional power contradict the claim that professions disinterestedly serve the public interest (see Chapter 5). Moreover the assertion that an extensive state apparatus has disseminated political power should be treated with caution. The devolution of decision making to DHAs in the 1982 reorganisation and the subsequent emphasis on devolution in the NHS reforms may lend support to these claims but it is possible to argue that stronger centralising forces have been at work (Paton, 1993).

If pluralism describes a competitive and meritocratic political world with access to policy making relatively open, Marxist and feminist accounts which relate to concepts such as elitism and corporatism conjure up very different impressions. Just as in the discussions of pluralism and neo-pluralism, what follows is a gross simplification of bodies of theory which are complex and varied. Orthodox *Marxist theory* is based on the premise that economic relations within capitalist systems determine which elements have control of the state and, ultimately, society. Capitalism is characterised by private ownership of wealth, which is concentrated in the hands of a class elite in society. Wealth is regenerated by using the labour of others to produce goods, payment for which (the wage) does not reflect the value added and profits thus accrue to the already powerful. This unacceptable situation is maintained by the execution of power in all its forms: for example, the coercive elements of state power such as the police, control of economic and social policy making and manipulation of the public consciousness through such institutions as the media and welfare institutions.

More recently Marxist writers, such as Poulantzas (1973) have revised this approach, rejecting the notion that the state is under the monopolistic control of a uniform elite. Society is not conceived as being made up of the capital-owning bourgeoisie and the proletariat alone, but contains other classes. Miliband (1969) argues that the state services the interests of the bourgeoisie; nevertheless, it has some autonomy and can act in the interests of the proletariat. To this end the state may produce policies which do not appear to benefit the capital-owning class but in effect, legitimise the status quo and aid capital accumulation. Applying this analysis to health care would lead one to conclude that the NHS, although partly responsible for the level of corporate taxation, exists to ameliorate the worst effects of capitalist modes of production on health (such as stress induced illness). Thus it maintains the relative productivity of the workforce as well as persuading workers of the good of the capitalist system. Similarly health and safety regulations may involve companies in expensive measures but these also contribute to a healthier workforce in the long term.

Feminism, like Marxism, offers several broad analyses of the state which can be grouped conventionally into liberal, Marxist and radical feminist accounts. Liberal feminists do not condemn the state as intrinsically patriarchal, but acknowledge both the dominance of men in positions of power within the state and the patriarchal nature of state policies. The traditional, unequal proportions of women holding office within government, the civil service or other public institutions are seen as problematic. The concern relates not only to unequal opportunities but also to the inability to influence state policies, the lack of which encourages the reproduction of gendered inequality. In contrast to liberal feminism, radical feminism extends the definition of politics to relationships of power within the private sphere. Accordingly radical feminism is somewhat silent on the role of the state other than to acknowledge its universal patriarchal nature. The analysis and strategies of radical feminism instead tend to concentrate on the interface between the state and men and women in a variety of private and unequal power relationships, rather than on the state and interest groups, or the position of women within the state.

Marxist–feminist accounts, as the term suggests, adopt the basic Marxist tenet that the state serves the interests of capital. Feminists such as Walby (1986) have criticised Marxism for its denial of capitalism's differential impact on men and women workers and for its inability to identify that the struggle for power in the capitalist state is gender as well as class related. Within this broad critique, some Marxist feminists focus on the nuclear family as functional for capitalism. An extension of Marxist–feminism proposes the inextricability of capitalism and patriarchy – each dependent on the other to endure (Eisenstein, cited by Walby, 1990). As Walby points out, this view tends to ignore the importance of patriarchy within the working class, when the latter in some Marxist accounts is seen as having some influence on state policies. These critical accounts have contributed to a view of the welfare state, including health care, which is variously employed in ensuring women's subordination to patriarchy or as the triumph of women's past struggles to improve welfare services (see Chapter 5).

Elite Theory and Alford's Typology

While Marxism and feminism both offer a view of the state reflecting a system of relations dominated by capitalism and/or patriarchy, they are more equivocal on the mechanism by which this is achieved. Some theorists from both traditions use elite theory to explain the process by which capitalism or patriarchy controls the state and policy making. Power, according to traditional elite theorists, is concentrated in a small section of society which, depending upon the state, may be constituted from the military, aristocracy, representatives of business or trade unions. As in Marxism, more recent approaches to elite theory suggest that different elites operate in separate spheres of influence.

Elite theory underpins Alford's (1975) classic study of health care planning in New York City, which analyses the relationships between three identified groups: the professional monopolists, the corporate rationalisers and the community. How readily each group is able to secure its interests depends upon the degree to which those interests correspond to the dominant structural interests of society, which in turn determine the way individual institutions operate. Although Alford's classification would encompass other occupations which exert a monopoly over certain work, such as physiotherapy or radiographers, doctors constitute the most important group of professional monopolists in health care. However doctors do not always have common interests: different specialisms may vie for territorial dominance within. Alford maintains that this potential for inner schism diminishes the ability of the profession to confront a common foe successfully.

The history of the NHS provides examples of this: internal differences in the medical profession occurred both at the inception of the NHS and in the 1975 junior hospital doctors' dispute (Klein, 1989). In addition, Hayward and Alaszewski's (1980) case study of the allocation of geriatric beds in a teaching district general hospital

(DGH) showed that some consultants were prepared to ditch support for colleagues. When a reduction in the total number of planned beds threatened the allocation to general medicine, support from the district medical team for the location of geriatric beds within the new DGH faded. On a much larger scale, the creation of fundholding has encouraged GPs to be more open in their criticism of the performance of colleagues in the trusts. However the nature of professional monopolists is such that, should something perceived as a common threat occur, for example the widespread registration of alternative therapists, the profession would forget internal differences and unite in common opposition.

The second most powerful group, the corporate rationalisers, also comprise differing occupations: government planners and public health agencies, managers of hospitals and medical schools. These are to be found within three broad organisational bases in the UK: the Department of Health, health authorities and provider institutions, such as hospital and community trusts. Alford suggested that the political culture and location are secondary to the group's main objective, which is to improve the delivery of health care. Corporate rationalisers respond to changes in the technology and organisation of health care. For example, it could be argued that the development of keyhole surgery and the leverage afforded by the purchaser–provider split in the NHS have prompted the active promotion of day surgery by corporate rationalisers.

In Alford's study the favoured method of dealing with possible conflicts over issues such as the improving of medical effectiveness was to discuss the issue in terms of abstract technicalities. Essentially this was a recourse to the rational method, which assumed that in a 'rational' world the various points of view could be accommodated and a 'best' solution would materialise. One would not have to look very far in past or present NHS activity to find evidence of this. From the mid 1970s the combination of a planning approach, which valued the use of extremely crude statistics about health care inputs, and consensus decision-making (see Chapter 3) seemed an attempt to approximate rational process. Pre-eminent corporate rationalisers in today's NHS, the public health doctors, also espouse a rational approach (see Chapter 6).

Alford wrote over two decades ago, in a period of US health care expansion and growing inflation. This was hitting hard those several groups of funders – the Federal government, insurance companies and corporate concerns – who provided health insurance for employees. They eventually brought pressure to bear on health care providers and the medical profession to slow down the rate of health care inflation, but it has been a difficult process. In the UK, the virtual state monopoly of health services and the central allocation of funds have produced more opportunities for rationalisation than the fragmented US system. In the past attempts by corporate rationalisers to reorientate health care in the NHS were weakened by the strength of the professional monopolists in the hospitals and the requirement to achieve consensus decisions. The purchaser–provider split in the NHS has weakened the position of hospital clinicians and strengthened the hand of the corporate rationalisers, who must now include GP fundholders in their number.

The third group identified by Alford, the community, is conceptualised within a US health care system where a considerable proportion of the population were – and still are – considered to be medically indigent. Alford cites examples of the urban poor as well as the lower middle class above the Medicaid income threshold. Their interests are repressed because institutional mechanisms within society are unsympathetic to their claims. The problem remains today. In the UK there is universal access to primary medical care (although dental and ophthalmic charges are now levied on some adults) and treatment is prescribed according to need rather than income and need. However inequities in service provision continue, as has the subordination of certain client groups' interests, such as those with learning disability or mental illness, to the demands of high technology medicine (Ham, 1992).

Changes have occurred since the 1970s. The critiques of the biomedical model and professional power and greater political activity by client interest groups such as MIND have, in Lukes' (1974) terms, articulated latent conflicts within health care. However, 'the community' rarely exists as a coherent entity, able to mobilise opinion, far less get a hearing. It is sometimes a more sensible strategy to make alliances. A local community may well combine with professional monopolists to prevent closure of a local hospital, but mobilising community views over a range of health issues is highly improbable. Consumer groups, acting as fragmented surrogates for community interests, may well be consulted by health authorities, but their views may not influence decisions. This is discussed further in Chapter 7.

Alford's typology is attractive in its simplicity and intuitive appeal; as such it has been used by several authors to interpret events in the NHS (Ham, 1981; Allsop, 1984; Harrison *et al.*, 1990; Wistow, 1992). While the particular application of Alford's framework was specific to the US – a health care system very different from the NHS now – the political divisions and pressures are to be found in all western states. With some adaptation and revision the model may help to clarify contemporary processes within the NHS. However it is reductionist and therefore somewhat undiscriminating in its approach. It does not cope very well with 'hybrid' groups within the NHS, such as doctors who manage clinical directorates, responsible for managerial decisions as well as their clinical practice. Had Alford's research been undertaken later, when the Reagan and Bush administrations sought to control spiralling health care costs, he might have considered the role of the state to be more important. As the NHS is a part of the state represented at the national and local level, studies of DHA policy making should acknowledge this as well as the politics of the local internal market. These intricacies perhaps call for more finely honed theories of interest group intermediation than those offered by Alford.

Policy Networks

Policy network theory examines the relationship between the state and groups who seek a role in policy making. It accepts the neo-pluralists' premise that the complexities of governing modern societies require a fragmentation of policy making. The state's role is perceived as variable, resulting in groups achieving differing degrees of access to policy making. To some extent this depends on the policy area, but the theory allows for discrimination between more or less successful groups within a network. Policy creation is not defined solely in terms of activity between a centralised government and interest group(s). A spider's web of relations, potentially encompassing government departments and local government as well as interest groups, can be accommodated by the theory.

As with any other mainstream political theory, policy network models have been the focus of debate and theoretical divergence, in part generated by the different political cultures of the USA and

Europe. For simplicity's sake this discussion will concentrate on the UK theoretical tradition, but a broader review of theoretical sources can be found in Rhodes and Marsh (1992a, 1992b). Within the UK literature there are differences of approach and terminology between, for example, the work of Rhodes and Marsh (1992a, 1992b) and that of Wilks and Wright (1987; see also Wright, 1988). Wilks and Wright, following in the tradition of the seminal research by Heclo and Wildavsky (1974) on the Treasury, place greater emphasis on the significance of informal relations and personal preferences in the study of political relationships between government and groups.

Policy networks theory acknowledges that the relationship between members of a network is based on reciprocity. The simplest resource which is used as currency is information. This, as Smith (1993) points out, may be as minimal as the government circulating information for comment, or, more extensively, high-powered discussions between government and interest group over detailed policy content.

Rhodes (1990) offers a typology of networks ranging from highly stable policy communities, which have a limited membership, to the loosely configured, somewhat conflictual issue networks. Professional networks, as the name indicates, are dominated by a professional group and represent professional interests. They are tightly knit and are insulated from other networks. Rhodes states that the NHS is the most frequently identified example of a professional network. Rhodes originally conceived of these and other categories of network as a continuum, but later conceded that this resulted in the blurring of two separate properties: the interests which dominate networks and the degree of integration, stability and exclusiveness of a network (Rhodes and Marsh, 1992a). The degree of stability and cohesion within a network depends upon members' perceptions of the gains accruing from the arrangement. Within policy communities, participants bring resources such as knowledge, influence or legitimacy. Groups in return gain influence in the policy-making process, which further enhances their status and power and the state gains co-operation in policy implementation. According to Rhodes (1988), however, the distribution of power within this symbiotic relationship is asymmetric. Ultimately the state's role in initiating policy secures for it the dominant position in a policy community. While there is some overlap between the concept of policy communities and corporatism, some perspectives within corporatist theory identify capture of the state by powerful interests.

Since there are significant advantages in stable relations to both state policy makers and interest groups (Jordan and Schubert, 1992), members of policy communities adhere to tacit 'rules of the game'. Groups holding unorthodox views which would destabilise the tightly knit community are excluded. Smith (1993) suggests that this action may not be conscious, but is reinforced by institutional structures and routines – constituting, in other words, a 'mobilisation of bias'. The lack of internal confrontation tends to depoliticise issues, and policy making thus becomes predictable. There are similarities between the above description of policy making in stable policy communities and the incrementalist politics identified by Lindblom (1979).

Policy communities do not exist in all areas of policy making but, where loosely configured and unstable issue networks prevail, policy outcomes are much less predictable, both in content and success of implementation. The political mêlée, which may well characterise such networks, results in policy inertia or policy change (Rhodes, 1988). Alternatively policy communities and issue networks may co-exist in the same policy area: an outer and inner ring of influence on policy making. Smith (1993) identifies a similar arrangement in the NHS, with the medical profession forming the core policy-making group with government (see Chapter 5).

Despite the advantages of stability conferred on the already power-ful members of policy communities (Rhodes and Marsh, 1992b; Jordan and Schubert, 1992; Smith, 1993), there is recognition that even the most inert of policy networks can change. Rhodes and Marsh (1992b) identify several external and internal catalysts of network change. International pressures can be disruptive, as can fluctuations in the domestic economy, technical advances or new knowledge about an issue. Rhodes and Marsh provide the example of the widely published research concerning the association between smoking and ill-health, which 'produced a major source of stress within the smoking network' (1992b: 194), phrasing which seems unintentionally evocative.

Possibly more significant than any of the agents noted so far is the influence of ideological change. As already noted, a shared system of beliefs may hold together policy communities, but beliefs are subject to reinterpretation. If, for example, the state as the more powerful member of policy community espouses a new ideology, the basis for a common approach to policy making may be destroyed if it conflicts with the beliefs or immediate interests of other members of the network. The influence of New Right ideas on the Conservative governments of the 1980s has both undermined professional power and changed the health policy agenda. This has challenged established policy networks, but the end result may not be as extreme as loosely configured issue networks operating at either central government or district health authority levels, since the government still requires the co-operation of the medical profession and the latter cannot afford to lose more influence over policy making.

Emphasis on the role of the state, which varies over time and in relation to the policy area, is the feature which most readily distinguishes the literature on policy networks from pluralist accounts of policy processes. In addition, networks theory breaks away from conceptual straitjackets which restrict pluralist analyses to observable displays of power and from the perception of stable and conservative state–elite interest group relationships portrayed by corporatist theory (Rhodes and Marsh, 1992a). Networks theory offers a more flexible framework for the analysis of policy making.

Simplifying the Complex

There are many more theories which attempt to offer an explanation of the policy process than those presented in this chapter. Even with the limited number described, making sense of where they fit in the scheme of things and deciding where they might best be applied is no simple matter. Part of the problem lies in the underlying rationale of the theory or model in question: some, such as those outlined by Lindblom (1959,1979) are more normative than others, while the work of Allison (1971), Alford (1975) and Rhodes (1988, 1990) seeks to explain rather than improve the policy-making process. Perhaps because of this difference in approach, some are more effective in policy analysis than others.

Observing what happens in a series of meetings within a DHA may produce the conclusion that decisions were apolitical and rational, or the product of SOPs (Allison, 1971), but these conclusions provide a picture of the decisional landscape rather than the underpinning of political interests. Hence a measured discussion which first establishes policy objectives and then, through careful and 'rational' analysis, produces satisfactory policy may well be symptomatic of a concentration of like-minded individuals, those with contradictory views having been excluded from the process. The work of Bachrach and Baratz (1970) and Lukes (1974) explains the mechanisms by which this is effected. For an understanding of which interests hold and benefit from power, we look to grand or meta-theories of state, such as Marxism, feminism and neo-pluralist accounts. However, even within these broad theoretical traditions, perceptions of the role of the state and its relationship with, for example, capitalism vary. For some Marxist authors the state, far from being controlled by capitalist classes, is relatively independent but sympathetic to the needs of capitalism. In contrast, neo-pluralists argue that power in liberal democracies is more widely dispersed among groups who defy rigid categorisation according to class or gender: for example, they cite the support of the medical profession for campaigns to control tobacco advertising, in opposition to powerful business interests.

Networks theory is located by some in the neo-pluralist tradition, but Smith (1993) asserts that the theory is sufficiently flexible to be used in association with a number of macro-theories ranging from Marxism, where exclusive policy-making networks would be controlled by capital interests, to pluralism in which loosely configured issue networks prevail and the state may respond to a number of interests. At the other end of the spectrum from state theories, the influence of informal and personal links between members of policy networks, highlighted by authors such as Wilks and Wright, may have much to offer small-scale analysis of the NHS.

From the Particular to the General

At one level it may be possible to apply a specific theory to events in the NHS, producing explanations which seem entirely plausible. The drawback is that the resulting analysis might ignore something of importance, simply because the theory is 'blind' to that aspect. If analysis moves one step back, some general questions emerge from the discussion of particular theories in this chapter which can be usefully applied to the contemporary NHS.

Is Policy Making Rational or Political?

The history of the National Health Service is replete with examples of attempts to introduce a more rational means of allocating scarce health resources. The planning system was introduced in 1976 in the hope that it would encourage, and permit the surveillance of, the Area Health Authorities' responses to government priorities. The initiative failed because it became bogged down in a cumbersome bureaucratic process and because local decisions had to be consensual. This meant they had to survive the medical profession's veto on health authority committees. Thus progress towards the objectives of central government, such as the movement of patients and resources into community care, was slow.

Since the early 1980s, changes within the NHS have introduced a managerial culture with a re-awakened commitment to rational processes and a focus on operational outcomes. Following the Griffiths Report (1983) the government ended consensus decision making and streamlined the management of the NHS, but perhaps the greatest potential stimulus to rational processes of decision making has been the development of internal markets. Health authorities are being urged by the NHSME to make use of their new found freedom to eschew incremental service development (NHSME, 1991a) and make 'rational changes' (NHSME, 1991b). They are also expected to note the views of GPs and 'the community'. This exhortation can be viewed in two ways: it may be taken to be a political process, in that consultation smooths the path for decisions, or could equally be considered a part of the information-gathering process which aids rational decision making. Nor should vigorous debate or uncontested decision making be assumed to indicate acquiescence in commissioning plans by all interested parties. Lukes reminds us that power is sometimes exercised in a covert manner.

Is Policy Making Radical or Incremental?

This apparently simple question needs to be dissected with care. It could be applied to the policy-making *process* which resulted in the NHS White Paper, *Working for Patients* (Department of Health, 1989). Alternatively, the word 'radical' might be used in relation to the potential *outcomes* of decision making within the internal market. Some suggest that times of crisis afford the right conditions for radical decision making, presumably on the basis that all concerned recognise that drastic circumstances call for drastic and often autocratic measures. During the Second World War the coalition government endorsed many policies which controlled the economy and restricted liberty in a way which would not be tolerated in peacetime. Did the perceived crisis in the NHS encourage and enable the small review group to adopt radical measures which bring the NHS closer to privatisation? Certainly the process, which excluded the medical profession from deliberations, was more radical than in the past.

Will the purchaser–provider split in health care produce more radical decisions in health care if health authorities are freed from the political pressures which encouraged traditional interpretations of health care, or is it more appropriate to think in terms of 'purposefully incremental' shifts in services? Local health service politics may have changed with the development of internal markets, but they have not disappeared. The enormity of the task for health authorities, inadequate knowledge about the cost and effectiveness of treatments and services and the constraints imposed by the market may limit the potential for change.

Who Has the Power?

It is impossible to get very far in either discussion of the questions outlined above without involving the concept of power. At one level the changes in the NHS from the early 1980s onwards have been to do with developing a more efficient and consumer-sensitive service, but more fundamentally they have been concerned with making a large section of the welfare state and the professionals who work within it more responsive to the broader agenda of central government. The increased control of the centre has been noted (Paton, 1993; Hood, 1991). It may be possible also to hypothesise crude shifts in power at the health authority level – in Alford's terms, from the professional monopolists to the corporate rationalisers and perhaps the community – but in some locations the internal market may have created powerful provider entities. These could manipulate the market and interpret the public interest in quite different terms, if they are permitted. The workings of the internal market, including the influence of fundholding and the ability of health authorities and ultimately the government to *manage* the market, are pivotal issues which will shape future health care in the UK.

The remaining chapters in this book are not concerned primarily with affirming the value of one particular policy-making theory over another, though they may point out where one is particularly illuminative. However they will reflect on the nature of power, which groups have power and the policy-making processes which result.

Bibliography

Alford, R. A. (1975) *The Politics of Health Care*, London: University of Chicago Press.

Allison, G. T. (1971) *Essence of Decision: Explaining the Cuban Missile Crisis*, Boston: Little, Brown.

Allsop, J. (1984) *Health Policy and the NHS*, London: Longman.

Bachrach, P. and Baratz, M. S. (1970) *Power and Poverty Theory and Practice*, London: Oxford University Press.

Butler, J. (1992) *Patients, Policies and Politics. Before and after Working for Patients*, Buckingham: Open University Press.

Department of Health (1989) *Working for Patients*, Cmnd 555, London: HMSO.

Dunleavy, P. (1981) 'Alternative theories of liberal democratic politics: the pluralist–marxist debate in the 1980s', in D. Potter with Anderson, J., Clarke, J. Coombes, P., Hall, S., Harris, L., Holloway, C. and Walton, T. (1981) *Society and the Social Sciences*, London: Routledge & Kegan Paul in association with the Open University Press.

Dunleavy, P. (1988) 'Theories of State in British Politics', in Drucker, H., Dunleavy, P., Gamble, A. and Peele, G. (1986), *Developments in British Politics*, rev. edn, London: Macmillan.

Eckstein, H. H. (1960) *The English Health Service: its origins, structure and achievements*, Cambridge, Mass.: Harvard University Press.

Ham, C. (1981) *Policy-making in the National Health Service. A case study of the Leeds Regional Hospital Board*, London: Macmillan.

Ham, C. (1992) *Health Policy in Britain*, 3rd edn, Basingstoke: Macmillan.

Ham, C. and Hill, M. (1993) *The Policy Process and the Modern Capitalist State*, 2nd edn, London: Harvester Wheatsheaf.

Harrison, S. (1988) *Managing the National Health Service – Shifting the Frontier?*, London: Chapman & Hall.

Harrison, S., Hunter, D. J. and Pollitt, C. (1990) *The Dynamics of British Health Policy*, London: Routledge.

Hayward, S. and Alaszewski, A. (1980) *Crisis in the Health Service. The politics of management*, London: Croom Helm.

Heclo, H. and Wildavsky, A. (1974) *The Private Government of Public Money*, London: Macmillan.

Hirst, P. (1987) 'Retrieving Pluralism', in W. Outhwaite and M. Mulkay (eds), *Social Theory and Social Criticism*, Oxford: Blackwell.

Hood, C. (1991) 'A public management for all seasons', *Public Administration*, vol. 69, Spring, pp. 3–19.

Hunter, D. J. (1980) *Coping with Uncertainty*, Letchworth: Research Studies Press.

Jacob, J. M. (1991) *Public Law*, Summer, pp. 255–81.

Jordan, G. and Schubert, K. (1992) 'A preliminary ordering of policy network labels', *European Journal of Political Research*, vol. 21, pp. 7–27.

Klein, R. (1989) *The Politics of the NHS*, 2nd edn, London: Longman.

Lindblom, C. E. (1959) 'The Science of Muddling Through', *Public Administration Review*, vol. 19, Spring, pp. 79–88.

Lindblom, C. E. (1979) 'Still Muddling, Not Yet Through', *Public Adminis-tration Review*, vol. 39, November/December, pp. 517–26.

Lindblom, C. E. and Woodhouse, E. J. (1993) *The Policy Making Process*, 3rd edn, Englewood Cliffs, NJ: Prentice-Hall.

Lukes, S. (1974) *Power: a radical view*, London: Macmillan.

McKeown, T. (1980) *The Role of Medicine: Dream, Mirage or Nemesis?*, 2nd edn, Oxford: Blackwell.

Miliband, R. (1969) *The State in Capitalist Society*, London: Weidenfeld & Nicolson.

Minogue, M., (1983) 'Theory and Practice in Public Policy and Adminis-tration', *Policy and Politics*, vol. 11, no. 1, pp. 63–8.

NHMSE (1991a) *Moving Forward – Needs, Services and Contracts*, London: Department of Health.

NHSME (1991b) *Purchasing Intelligence*, London: Department of Health.

Paton, C. (1993) 'Devolution and Centralism in the National Health Service', *Social Policy and Administration*, vol. 27, no. 2, pp. 83–108.

Poulantzas, N. (1973) *Political Power and Social Classes*, London: New Left Books.

Rhodes, R. A. W. (1988) *Beyond Westminster and Whitehall*, London: Unwin Hyman.

Rhodes, R. A. W. (1990) 'Policy Networks. A British Perspective', *Journal of Theoretical Politics*, vol. 2, no. 3, pp. 293–317.

Rhodes, R. A. W. and Marsh, D. (1992a) 'Policy Networks in British Politics. A critique of existing approaches', in D. Marsh and R. A. W. Rhodes (eds), *Policy Networks in British Government*, Oxford: Oxford University Press.

Rhodes, R. A. W. and Marsh, D. (1992b) 'New Directions in the study of policy networks', *European Journal of Political Research*, vol. 21, pp. 181–205.

Smith, M. J. (1990) 'Pluralism, reformed pluralism and neopluralism: the role of pressure groups in policy-making,' *Political Studies*, vol. 38, pp. 302–22.

Smith, M. J. (1993) *Pressure, Power and Policy, State Autonomy and Policy Networks in Britain and the United States*, London: Harvester Wheatsheaf.

Walby, S. (1986) *Patriarchy at work: patriarchal and capitalist relations in employ-ment*, Cambridge: Polity Press.

Walby, S. (1990) *Theorizing Patriarchy*, Oxford: Blackwell.

Wilks, S. and Wright, M. (1987) *Comparative Government–Industry Relations*, Oxford: Clarendon Press.

Willcocks, A. J. (1967) *The Creation of the National Health Service*, London: Routledge & Kegan Paul.

Wistow, G. (1992) 'The Health Service Policy Community', in D. Marsh and R. A. W. Rhodes (eds), *Policy Networks in British Government*, Oxford: Oxford University Press.

Wright, M. (1988) 'Policy Community, Policy Network and Comparative Industrial Policies', *Political Studies*, vol. 36, pp. 593–612.

3
Health Care Models and Welfare Themes

Ian Kendall

This chapter provides an overview of changes in health care in Britain since the first part of the nineteenth century. The knowledge and practices of health care practitioners have changed dramatically in this period. Most forms of medical intervention that we take for granted towards the end of the twentieth century were unknown at the beginning of the nineteenth century. Not only have forms of health care changed but the role of the state in health care has also been transformed in this period. This transformation can be said to exemplify what is often referred to as 'the development of the welfare state'. Health care in Britain in the middle of the nineteenth century and health care in Britain in the middle of the twentieth century serve as classic examples of contrasting models of state welfare. For much of the nineteenth century the dominant model of state welfare was the residual model – a minimal state model of health care. By the middle of the twentieth century the dominant model of state welfare was the institutional model – a universalist/citizenship model of health care. This chapter will provide an overview of the changes involved in the move from the minimal state model to the universalist/citizenship model with particular reference to the arrangements for organising and financing health care. The resulting account provides not only a historical context to the present-day debates addressed in the remaining chapters but also examples of the welfare perspectives and policy making processes identified in Chapters 1 and 2.

A Minimal State Model of Health Care

At the beginning of the nineteenth century in the UK there was a local system of public assistance for the destitute, based on parishes (the Poor Law). Insofar as ill-health was either a cause or consequence of such destitution, there was some rudimentary care of sick people as part of this provision. The aims of the Poor Law included the expenditure of minimal sums of public money to achieve broader social and political goals of the sort that subsequent Marxist analyses would identify with modern 'welfare states', notably social and political control.

The Poor Law was 'reformed' in 1834 following the well-known policy process of a Royal Commission leading to an Act of Parliament (Poor Law Amendment Act, 1834). The 'New Poor Law' (post-1834) has been widely identified with the economic liberal strand of the 'political right' perspective. Its core ideas included notions of individualistic freedom and self-help, and were essentially antithetical to anything more than minimal state intervention in areas broadly encompassed by the categories of economic and social policy. The 1834 legislation was intended to proscribe the role of public assistance by a more precise delineation of who might be in receipt of such assistance. This was to be achieved through a policy of 'indoor relief' and the 'workhouse test'. 'Indoor relief' involved the poor law authorities providing relief only within an institutional setting: individuals and families would have to live in the workhouse in order to receive support. The 'workhouse test' involved ensuring that conditions in the workhouse were obviously less attractive than those which would be afforded to the lowest paid worker living outside the workhouse. The 'workhouse test' would act as an effective and clearly intended deterrent to all but the most desperate and destitute of individuals. Only those in the greatest need would present themselves to the Poor Law authorities. The welfare role of the state and associated public expenditures, including any health care provision by the state, would be minimal.

Non-state Health Care

The potential to maintain this minimal state model of health care would be facilitated by effective and extensive health care located in the non-state sector. During the nineteenth century non-state, especially voluntary, institutions appeared well placed to meet the health care needs of the nation with limited recourse to state intervention. Philanthropic, charitable activity was represented by the voluntary hospitals. A working-class mutual aid tradition was represented by the Friendly Societies. Membership of the latter grew throughout the nineteenth century. They were the largest exclusively working-class organisations in Britain and most of them provided medical benefit – principally the payment of sickness benefit and the services of general practitioners under contract to provide medical services to their members.

Beyond the Minimal State Model of Health Care

Contrary to the aims and aspirations associated with the New Poor Law, the state in Britain was significantly involved in health care provision by the outbreak of the First World War, in 1914. This came about in a number of ways, some in an incrementalist fashion, others as a result of relatively radical policy innovations. All might be seen as at least in part the product of political expediency.

Given the relatively limited powers of the relevant central authority (The Poor Law Commission) there was ample opportunity for local variations in the operation of the New Poor Law, including the operationalisation of 'indoor relief'. Many individuals continued to be maintained by the poor law authorities beyond the confines of the workhouse via 'outdoor relief'. This provides an early example of the difficulty of ensuring equity and consistency of treatment in locally managed services. However regardless of the fiscal or ideological preferences of local 'Poor Law' managers, the concept of 'indoor relief' was anyway virtually impossible to sustain in the new industrial, urban centres of population in the face of localised rises in unemployment: there was insufficient space in the workhouse to accommodate all those that the poor law authorities deemed in need of some form of assistance.

Industrialisation and urbanisation also contributed to another extension of state activity in health matters. This was the 'public health question' linked to the increasingly well documented health problems associated especially with new industrial towns. Given the enactment of public health legislation following statistical representations of the public health problem, we might presume that this represented a model of rational decision making, but it is doubtful that this model could accommodate the considerable delay in getting effective public health legislation on the statute book. The marked difference between death rates in urban and rural areas was being documented by the Registrar-General in the 1830s, but almost a quarter of a century would pass before a really effective piece of public health legislation was placed on the statute book (Thane, 1982: 40). The delay might be explained partly by the continuing dominance of the beliefs and ideas that sustained the minimal state model of health care, and by the power of those who had vested interests in low levels of local taxation and/or the provision of water and sewerage systems only to those who could afford to pay the market price for such services.

The recognition of the need to respond in some way to public health issues provided the basis for further extensions beyond the minimal state model of health care. Under section 37 of the Sanitary Act, 1866, local authorities were empowered to build their own hospitals and by 1900 there would be nearly one thousand isolation hospitals and other institutions as part of the local government public health service. Local government was now a provider of public and personal health services, the latter being further extended in 1906 when local government acquired the powers to develop school medical services and health visiting services.

Why did local government hospitals have to be built in response to the public health problem when there was already a well-established voluntary hospital tradition? This reflects in part the limitations of voluntary hospital provision. It was a general feature of charity in nineteenth century Britain that it was highly localised (Thane, 1982: 21) and this was true of the voluntary hospitals. The range and scope of their provision was linked to the range and scope of private practice in an area, for it was from the latter that their doctors obtained their major remuneration. As well as this significant spatial limitation, 'the voluntary movement never became more than marginally involved in the needs of the chronically sick' (Pinker, 1966: 72), who constituted 'less interesting' cases for purposes of teaching and research, and to which little or no professional prestige attached (Abel-Smith, 1964: 45).

The outcome was that the state assumed a responsibility for what was left undone by charity and private enterprise (Thane, 1982: 41).

The epidemics associated with urbanisation and the restricted scope of voluntary hospital activity led not only to the development of local government hospitals, but also to an extension of the health care activities of the poor law authorities as the latter became the custodians and carers of large numbers of sick paupers. One response by the poor law authorities was to create not only separate 'wards for the sick' in the workhouse, but also separate poor law infirmaries. The latter were soon being identified as 'the real hospitals of the land' in *The Lancet Commission Report* (quoted in Abel-Smith, 1964: 50).

The development of this Poor Law medical service occurred with little or no specific legislation being passed to extend the duties of the Poor Law authorities. The changes attest to the potential significance of incrementalist change in social policy and to the role of professionals in redefining the scope and nature of a 'public service' (Brand, 1965; Hodgkinson, 1967). Although these Poor Law medical services were of variable and often minimal quality, nonetheless a further state involvement in health care was emerging that went beyond the minimal state model of health care.

Like the voluntary hospitals, Friendly Society health care also had its limitations. Membership of the societies was associated with the better off members of the working class and few societies admitted both men and women. Most women earned too little to pay their own contributions and few working-class families could afford double contributions (Thane, 1982: 29, 30). The health care needs of those unable to afford Friendly Society membership would often be met by the Poor Law infirmaries and dispensaries that were the major providers of health care for women, children and older people – an early indication of the importance of implications of state welfare activities for social divisions associated with age and gender.

Some of the limitations of Friendly Society health care were addressed by one of the more explicit and radical policy changes introduced before the NHS itself. This was the introduction of the social insurance model of state health care in a scheme to which the label 'National Health Insurance' (NHI) was attached as part of the National Insurance Act, 1911. Essentially this involved a transition common to a number of European countries, in which voluntary health insurance developed by working-class mutual aid societies forms the basis of a state-regulated system of compulsory health insurance. By this means the medical benefits associated with voluntary health insurance are extended to a larger proportion of the population. The system of employee contributions is maintained (although now as part of a state scheme) with additional resources coming from employer contributions and general tax revenues.

When public health legislation is put alongside the local government hospitals, the Poor Law Medical Service and the establishment of NHI, we can identify a significant change in the role of the state in health care between the beginning of the nineteenth century and the beginning of the First World War. The relative roles of state and non-state institutions in health care were changing and it could be argued that these changing roles indicated a degree of (possibly reluctant) acceptance of key elements of the social democratic arguments relating to the inefficiencies and injustices of unregulated markets in socially important goods such as health care.

NHI was introduced in the same period as a range of other health and welfare reforms by a 'left of centre' Liberal government. These reforms can be readily understood from a Marxist perspective, given the extent to which some of them – for example, the development of health visiting and school health services – were in line with concerns about 'national efficiency', that is the economic and military effectiveness of a major capitalist society. The limitations of these reforms would also be readily understandable from a feminist perspective when we note that the introduction of a social insurance based, limited health service (NHI) excluded not only hospital care but also GP provision for men in non-manual occupations, all children and most working-class women. This social insurance scheme also provided an excellent case study of the impact of professional power and influence on health care policy making. However, whereas previous developments (public health and the Poor Law medical services) drew significant support from members of the medical profession, on this occasion there was conflict between a 'reformist' (Liberal) government and professional associations (principally the British Medical Association – BMA) over the terms and conditions under which general practitioners would work as part of the new National Health Insurance scheme.

The Politics of NHI Organisation

The politics of NHI were difficult for the Liberal government as the reform would have an impact on potentially powerful interest groups whose circumstances – especially financial circumstances – might be adversely affected by the introduction of the new scheme. These groups constituted an 'issue network' (see Chapter 2) and included the doctors and the Friendly Societies. A state social insurance scheme appeared to pose a very real threat to the latter as providers of voluntary health insurance. Their opposition was contained by enabling them to administer the government's scheme as approved societies. But the political and administrative advantages of this manoeuvre merely brought the government into conflict with the medical profession and the industrial insurance companies. The former were opposed to being permanently consigned to the control of Friendly Societies in a government health scheme: this was seen by the profession as involving a significant degree of lay control and a real threat to clinical freedom (professional autonomy). The latter saw their lucrative insurance business threatened by the potential expansion of their competitors as part of a government scheme. In the end the conflict was contained by two managerial and administrative devices.

Firstly, the requirements for the 'approved societies', which were responsible for the day-to-day management of NHI, were constructed in such a way that industrial insurance companies, in addition to Friendly Societies, could qualify to administer the scheme on behalf of the government. Secondly, a system for contracting with and paying the GPs was devised that avoided direct control by the approved societies.

The politics of NHI serves as perhaps the first example of a recurrent theme in which the detailed arrangements of health care reforms are significantly restructured to accommodate the perceived interests of key groups. It also represented a major exercise in what was later to be categorised as welfare pluralism, given that the day-to-day administration and delivery of NHI benefits was effectively 'contracted out' to self-employed professionals (GPs) and what we would now call the independent sector (Friendly Societies and insurance companies).

Towards a Universalist/Citizenship Model of Health Care

The inter-war years saw incremental developments in state intervention in health care in two directions. Firstly, access to general practitioner services under NHI was extended; secondly, the basis of an embryonic local government health service was discernible by the 1930s, by which time local authorities had an obligation to provide, or at least finance, an adequate midwifery service and the power to provide a home help service. Both these services were often provided by grants to relevant voluntary organisations, a further example of welfare pluralism.

Local government also became a major provider of hospital care. Local authorities had inherited hospitals built by the nineteenth century sanitary authorities. There were further piecemeal additions to this stock of fever hospitals and other sanatoria and, following the Mental Treatment Act, 1930, the local authority asylums had been redesignated as mental hospitals. But the most significant change had been the Local Government Act, 1929. This Act left the Poor Law on the statute book, but abolished the Poor Law authorities (Boards of Guardians) and transferred all powers, duties, buildings, personnel and responsibility for 'paupers' to county councils and county boroughs. The result was the potential for the establishment of a general municipal *hospital* service. Indeed, with the other services mentioned above (such as home helps and midwifery), there was considerable scope for the development of a more comprehensive and co-ordinated set of municipal *health services*. Although few local authorities exploited these opportunities in the 1930s, the circumstances were a model scenario for further modest, incremental extensions of state intervention in health care via both National Health Insurance and local government in line with any perceived pressure in that direction from the electorate.

While further expansion of Poor Law hospital services and their incorporation into local government complemented the acute focus of the voluntary hospitals, the latter were finding it increasingly difficult to meet needs even within their own narrowly defined sphere of competence. Medical advances were increasingly associated with escalating medical costs, indicating a seemingly inevitable conflict between the scope of voluntary contributions and charitable bequests on the one hand and the needs of modern hospital services on the other. These escalating costs associated with advances in medical technology were taking the voluntary hospitals up to and beyond the limits of philanthropy. It was no longer possible to sustain the standards of hospital work associated with the most eminent institutions without recourse to a much more substantial reliance on patient charges, some form of government funding or a combination of the two.

Alongside the incremental changes in National Health Insurance and local government, and the crises in the costs and character of the voluntary hospital sector, there is clear evidence that by the 1930s the issue of health care reform was on the political agenda and not just a matter of private debate between the health care professionals and the existing health care institutions. A series of reports and associated recommendations emerged from a variety of sources throughout the inter-war period.

One consistent theme was the need for a rationalisation of the fragmented and somewhat haphazard assemblage of health care institutions that constituted pre-NHS health care in the UK. A partial National Health Insurance scheme that excluded children, non-earning wives, the self-employed, many old people and higher paid employees operated alongside other services whose scope and effectiveness depended on such vagaries as the wealth of each area and the political initiative of different local authorities. This situation was a source of considerable inefficiencies associated with the duplication and lack of co-ordination of staff and facilities. These arrangements also provided ample opportunity for enormous variations in service provision in different parts of the country. The overall effect was of profound regional disparities, as indicated by per capita measurements of GPs, consultants and hospital beds.

The perceived inefficiencies of the hospital sector of the health services were a focus of governmental concern with Britain's involvement in the Second World War, beginning in 1939. This was related in part to planning for the expected significant civilian air raid casualties. The solution to the haphazard and extremely variable quality of existing hospital services was their temporary nationalisation in the form of the Emergency Medical Services. The result was extensive investment to bring the poorest quality institutions up to a reasonable standard. This experience added weight to the arguments that existing provision was both inefficient and inequitable.

In October 1941 the Ministry of Health announced that the government was committed to establishing a comprehensive *hospital* service after the war, including the intention that appropriate treatment should be available to all who needed it – the first clear cut government commitment to the principle of universality. The more significant advocacy of this principle came in December 1942 with the publication of the Beveridge Report which included a recommendation that, after the war, Britain should have not just a comprehensive *hospital* service, but a comprehensive *health* service. The Report recommended the 'separation of medical treatment from the administration of cash benefits and the setting up of a comprehensive medical service for every citizen, covering all treatment and every form of disability under the supervision of the Health Departments' (Beveridge, 1942: 48, para. 106).

The social insurance principle, introduced amid considerable political conflict in 1911, was to be abandoned for health care. If a modern health care system could not be maintained by philanthropic activity it should, according to Beveridge, be maintained by public expenditure (taxation) rather than private expenditure (service user charges and private insurance). If implemented by the government the Beveridge principles would represent the final stage in a transition from a minimal state model of health care to a universalist/citizenship model of health care.

The Politics of NHS Organisation

In February 1943 the House of Commons debated the Beveridge Report. The government announced that it welcomed the conception of a reorganised and comprehensive health service which would cover the people as a whole. The subsequent policy-making process had similarities with that leading to the establishment of the NHI. The medical profession had contributed to placing health care reform on the pre-war agenda and the profession's own wartime experiences reinforced a considerable professional commitment to reform. But with the publication of the Beveridge Report and the wartime government's commitment to a NHS, considerable professional attention would be directed to securing the best interests of the doctors. The result was considerable conflict between the profession's representatives, including the BMA, and successive Ministers of Health in the Coalition and Labour governments.

The Coalition government's first attempt to take forward the process of reform was the never officially published 'Brown Plan', named after the then Minister of Health. It drew on the pre-war significance of municipal health services with a proposal for a unified health service based on regional local government units. The voluntary hospitals would be utilised (and therefore at least partially financed) by the new service, but would not be nationalised. GPs would be employed in a full-time salaried service. The Plan was discussed with interested parties but was clearly opposed by the BMA. In December 1943 a new Minister of Health, Henry Willink, was appointed.

In February 1944 the first official publication emerged. This was *A National Health Service* (Ministry of Health, 1944), which proposed a local organisation for the new service based on joint local authority areas. The new organisation would take over municipal hospitals and lay down the conditions under which voluntary hospitals would participate, in return for which they would receive grants towards part of the cost of patient care. Under this scheme the GPs would be under contract to a Central Medical Board, with remuneration in the same format as the NHI. However doctors working in health centres would be salaried and the central Board was to have the power to refuse doctors the right to practise in over-doctored areas and to compel new doctors to work in poorly-served areas. The BMA was still not satisfied with the government proposals, especially any form of salaried service for GPs, the direction of doctors and the significant role for local government. The medical profession's antagonism towards local government was proving a major impediment to reaching agreement. The parallels with the conflict over NHI were clear: local government, like the Friendly Societies before 1911, represented a significant degree of lay control and interference with professional autonomy.

By the early summer of 1945 the minister had assembled the elements of an alternative plan (the Willink Plan). This introduced a two tier system of regional and area planning authorities made up of equal local authority and voluntary hospital representation. Municipal hospitals would remain under local government control. Health centres were relegated to 'experimental status' and the powers of direction previously proposed for the Central Board would disappear. Local administration of GP services would be undertaken by a modified version of the existing NHI committees. Although representatives of the medical profession were said to be more supportive of the Willink Plan, it was never officially published. The 1945 General Election led to an overwhelming victory for the Labour Party and there was a new Minister of Health – Aneurin Bevan.

Bevan's solution to the conflicts was to manage the GP services through a model based on the existing political compromises of NHI (GPs would remain independent, self-employed contractors) and to circumvent the issue of local government control by nationalising the municipal and voluntary hospitals. The resulting characteristics of the new NHS included the following. Firstly, the service would be funded by national government with revenue derived from predominantly national rather than local taxation; within the former, social insurance contributions (National Insurance) would play only a limited role and would in no way determine entitlements to use the NHS. Secondly, and related to the financial arrangements, there would be only a limited role for local government in providing health care (for example, community nursing services) and employing doctors (such as Medical Officers of Health). Rather than uniting the service around the 'embryonic municipal health service' a tripartite organisational structure was established with separate organisational and financial arrangements for the hospital services, the GP services and those community and other health services (such as ambulances) that remained within local government. A major and very popular component of the post-war state welfare would remain profoundly undemocratic in its organisational arrangements. Finally, for doctors and their patients there would be the doctor of choice, free treatment at the point of use and referral to the hospital by general practitioners.

As with the introduction of NHI, we know that sections of the medical profession were active as pressure groups; we know that the plans for the health service changed with regard to administrative and financial arrangements and that the plans changed in ways which can be seen to benefit the sections of the medical profession. This is most obvious with the role of local government in health care which was significantly diminished when both voluntary and municipal hospitals were nationalised. The democratic and bureaucratic challenge to professional autonomy represented by local government was eliminated. Furthermore, the nationalised hospital system would inherit a management system much more like that of the voluntary than the municipal hospital system, one that placed considerable emphasis on clinical freedom. In addition, the most prestigious hospitals – the teaching hospitals – were afforded a special administrative and financial status within the NHS. They were to be financed directly by the ministry, enabled to retain their pre-NHS endowments and given considerable managerial autonomy. Once again the political process associated with a major health care reform culminated in a conflict between a 'reformist' (Labour) government and professional associations (principally the BMA) over what might be regarded as essentially organisational issues.

The establishment of the NHS was also similar to the establishment of NHI in forming part of a wider set of social policy reforms introduced by the wartime Coalition and the post-war Labour governments – especially the latter. These included secondary education for all, universalist social security policies (following the Beveridge Report, 1942), housing and town planning legislation and a new Children's Act. As well as representing the operationalising of social democratic perspectives on welfare, these changes can be interpreted from a Marxist perspective as a further accommodation between capital and labour. They certainly represent a dramatic change in the relative roles of state and voluntary institutions in health care by comparison with the situation one hundred years earlier. The state was now ostensibly committed to the universalist/citizenship model of health care.

The Universalist/Citizenship Model of Health Care

Essentially this model presumes the necessity and desirability of a major role for the state in relation to providing resources for health care. This health care will be available on a universalist basis: that is, all members of society will be able to use the state health services. Entitlement will based on citizenship rather than either membership of and contributions to a social insurance scheme (NHI) or identification as poor through a test of means.

Given the concerns voiced about pre-war health services it is unsurprising that the new NHS was seen as the means to provide a more efficient and equitable health service. One means of getting a more efficient health service would be through 'rational planning'; the potential of which had been indicated by the arrangements put in place during the Second World War. There was evidence of planning in the NHS, most obviously with the publication of the Hospital Plan in 1962. This was intended to provide 'a rational basis for the development of the hospital services' (Allsop, 1984: 55) but the significant investment proposed for London, especially the London teaching hospitals, was simply the 'cheapest' way, in the short run, to remedy deficiencies in medical education (see Abel-Smith, 1990: 13). The plan was 'rational' for short-term goals relating to medical manpower and 'rational' in relation to a particular perspective on hospital provision (it introduced the concept of the District General Hospital) but 'less rational' for those who saw a continuing role for small community hospitals (most small hospitals would go when the new District General Hospitals were in place).

It was also far from clear that the plan represented 'rational planning' for the NHS as a whole, especially for those concerned about the interrelationship between hospital and community health services, notably policies of community care for people with mental health problems. Government commitment to the latter was reasonably clear following the Mental Health Act, 1959. The Hospital Plan took the commitment a stage further with a planned major reduction of mental hospital in-patient facilities. But when the supposedly complementary health and welfare plans were published in the following year it was far from clear that local government would develop an appropriate response in terms of new community mental health services.

The limitations and problems of planning might be explained by the political conflicts involved in establishing the NHS and especially the political compromise of the tripartite organisational structure of the service. This separation of hospital from community health services provided the rationale for producing separate plans for the two sectors despite their symbiotic relationship; the third part of the tripartite structure involved the GPs and their independent contractor status made it more difficult to plan their services. The political compromise of 1948 gave every appearance of hindering rather than helping the planning process.

Nor did the continuing problems of cost escalation encourage governments to engage in 'rational planning'. Demographic trends, medical advances and rising expectations increased the potential volume of treatable illness confronting the NHS and successive governments found themselves confronting a situation in which additional expenditure was necessary merely to enable the NHS to maintain the existing range and standard of provision. The first major report on the working of the NHS commissioned by the 1951–5 Conservative government was concerned about its 'present and prospective cost' and how to limit 'the burden on the Exchequer'

(Guillebaud, 1956). It was apparent that containing the costs of the new NHS was firmly on the political agenda, and probably higher up that agenda than planning the new NHS. At the same time, critics from a New Right perspective were swift to point to the 'public burden' of the NHS as evidence of the errors of the social democratic perspective. In the process they seemed conveniently to forget the financial problems that had beset voluntary hospitals in the pre-war era (and indeed Friendly Societies before the introduction of NHI) and the substantial wartime public investment that had been necessary to bring much of Britain's hospital services up to a tolerable standard.

The pursuit of a more equitable allocation of health care resources was one of the more clearly stated goals of the service (Klein, 1983: 25). The key inequalities concerned the allocation of, access to and the utilisation of the resources and facilities of the NHS. The service's inheritance was one of profound spatial inequalities with a set of associated inequalities linked to social class. Also part of the inheritance, especially linked to the different histories of the voluntary and local government (Poor Law) hospitals, was the different provision for different types of care, different groups of patient and different sorts of need.

It was hoped that the elimination of explicit financial barriers (user charges) to the utilisation of health care would have a profound impact on social class inequalities in utilisation and, by implication, on social class inequalities in health. However by the mid-1960s there was a growing recognition that the 'higher income groups know how to make better use of the Service' (Titmuss, 1968: 196). The 'free play of market forces' may have been significantly moderated with the introduction of a largely 'free at the point of consumption' universalist health service, but the 'free play of social forces' (Pinker, 1971) generated persistent evidence of the ability of some social groups to make more effective use of the NHS.

Inequalities also persisted as a consequence of the already identified limitations of post-war planning. Resources were allocated on the basis of historic cost-budgeting ensuring that all areas benefited from increasing resources, but perpetuating the inherited pattern of inequalities. In addition, the types of care and patient who were eventually identified as the 'Cinderella areas' of the NHS – mental health services, elderly people and people with learning difficulties – represented those areas of medical and nursing activity to which the professions attached the lowest status. These distinctions were long-established and were clear before the twentieth century when a higher status was accorded to voluntary hospital staff and patients.

It was also becoming increasingly apparent that the relationship between social and economic factors and the utilisation of health care, and between health care and health status was a complex one. Seeking to provide good quality health care on a universalist basis at little or no cost to service users did not translate simply into either equitable utilisation of that health care or reduced inequalities in health. Finally we should note the significance of the organisational structure of the NHS. It was an obstacle to planning for a more equitable service and was a particular problem in relation to monitoring inequalities linked to location (territorial injustices), requiring the collection, collation and analysis of the separate resource allocation figures for the hospital service, for the local authority community health services and for general practitioner services. The 'Cinderella areas' were especially vulnerable particularly in relation to the growing commitment to community care. The 'easier task' (in resource terms) of running down old-fashioned hospital provision (such as the old asylums) rested with one part of the tripartite structure while the 'more difficult task' of expanding new community based services rested with the other two parts of that structure. In addition limited mechanisms were in place to co-ordinate the latter two (GPs and local authority community health services).

Politics of NHS Reorganisation

By the 1960s it was possible to make a case for organisational reform based on identifiable trends in practice and policy initiatives; these included early discharge schemes in the maternity services, the attachment of nursing staff to general practice and the commitment to developing community-based mental health services (Abel-Smith, 1978: 35–7). In the event, 12 years would pass before the service was reorganised – a time-scale that was at least partly indicative of the continuing political sensitivity surrounding organisational issues in health care, especially the professional interests involved.

When the Labour government (1964–70) made its first pronouncements on a possible organisational restructuring in health care in what became known as the First Green Paper (Ministry of Health,

1968), it had already set in train parallel reviews to restructure the personal social services and local government. The first tangible contradiction to emerge from this process was the Seebohm Committee recommendation for a different division between health and social care in which key services located in the local authority health departments would move to a new local authority social services department rather than the new Area Health Boards (Seebohm, 1968).

Before publishing a Second Green Paper in 1970 the government reassured the medical profession that the 'new NHS' would not be part of the 'new local government' and took steps to implement most of the recommendations of the Seebohm Committee to the evident satisfaction of most of the social work profession. The Second Green Paper (DHSS, 1970) confirmed that new Area Health Authorities (AHAs) would be outside local government, but there would be enhanced potential for NHS/local government co-operation through coterminosity: the boundaries of the new AHAs would match the boundaries of the new local authorities proposed by the Redcliffe-Maud Commission. Finally it proposed a means to resolve the questions relating to the division of services between the new Social Services Departments and the new Area Health Authorities: for example, which agency should run the home help service? The proposal was that all that was social work related would remain in local government as part of the new Social Services Department. All that was medical and nursing-related was to move outside local government, into the reorganised NHS (DHSS, 1970: 10, para. 31). Before the reorganisations were finally implemented in 1974 further documents were published by what was now a Conservative government (1970–74). A Consultative Document (May 1971) and a White Paper (August 1972) set out the government's proposals for England, with separate documents setting out the similar proposals for Wales and Scotland. Crucially a set of regional health authorities (RHAs) were reintroduced in a direct line relationship between the Secretary of State and the AHAs (see DHSS, 1971, 1972).

Since the First Green Paper was published in 1968 a combination of medical politics and party politics (in the form of a change of government) had extended the process of reorganisation over a period of six years. This was indicative of the extent to which the organisational arrangements for health care continued to generate considerable conflict and hostility. As with the proposals for NHI and the NHS, the final outcome bore limited resemblance to the original proposals as separate arrangements for general practitioner and regional authorities found their way back into the organisational structure and local government involvement in health care, rather than being significantly enhanced (First Green Paper), was dramatically diminished (by the Second Green Paper). Local health services would be linked with local democracy only through the tenuous device of local authority representation on the health authorities and the minimal participation of citizens in Community Health Councils. Some aspects of the old tripartite division disappeared, most obviously between hospital and community-based nursing services, but a new and even clearer health and social care division was being established following the principle of dividing these services in relation to their links with health or social work professionals. Indeed the outcome of the 1974 reorganisation was a more clearly delineated administrative, financial and professional division between health and social care than had existed at any previous stage in the history of post-war health and community care policies (Carrier and Kendall, 1995: 17). It was another political compromise and would attract a good deal of criticism for the rest of the 1970s.

Royal Commission on NHS

The first major government publication on health care in 1979 was that of the Royal Commission. This had been set up by the 1974–79 Labour government, but reported to a newly elected Conservative government. The Commission endorsed many of the criticisms which had been directed at the 1974 reorganisation, concluding that they could recommend 'no simple, universal panacea for the cure of the administrative ills of the NHS' (Merrison, 1979: 325). Perhaps more significantly the Commission lent considerable support to the concept of a National Health Service and to the basic priorities of the service. The Commission's brief had included the examination of the possibility of a greater reliance on insurance and charges as a means of financing the NHS. It rejected both, emphasising a point which was to be made with considerable force over the next decade, that by comparison with the health care systems of other advanced industrial societies, the NHS was remarkably cheap and by implication probably quite efficient.

The 1979 Royal Commission was in all crucial respects a whole-hearted endorsement of the universalist/citizenship model of health care and of the arguments identified with the social democratic perspective. It stands in marked contrast to the Royal Commission produced almost a century and half previously and which had equally whole-heartedly endorsed the minimal state model of health care and ushered in the New Poor Law. A range of economic, political and social factors eroded the principles endorsed by the Royal Commission of 1834. The chapters that follow will give an indication of the current state of the principles endorsed by the Royal Commission of 1979.

Bibliography

Abel-Smith, B. (1964) *The Hospitals 1800–1948: a study in social administration in England and Wales*, London: Heinemann.

Abel-Smith, B. (1978) *National Health Service: the first thirty years*, London: HMSO.

Abel-Smith, B. (1990) 'The first forty years', in J. Carrier and I. Kendall (eds), *Socialism and the NHS*, Aldershot: Gower.

Allsop, J. (1984) *Health Policy and the National Health Service*, London: Longman.

Beveridge, W. (1942) *Report: Social Insurance and Allied Services*, Cmd 6404, London: HMSO.

Black, D. (1980) *Inequalities in Health: Report of a Research Working Party*, London: DHSS.

Brand, J. (1965) *Doctors and the State*, Baltimore, MD: Johns Hopkins Press.

Carrier, J. and Kendall, I. (1990) 'Working for patients?', in J. Carrier and I. Kendall (eds), *Socialism and the NHS: Fabian Essays in Health Care*, Gower: Aldershot

Carrier, J. and Kendall, I. (1994) 'Professionalism and inter-professionalism in health and community care: some theoretical issues', in J. Carrier, P. Owens and J. Horder (eds), *Interprofessional issues in Community and Primary Health Care*, London: Macmillan.

DHSS (1970) *The Future Structure of the National Health Service*, Second Green Paper, London: HMSO.

DHSS (1971) *National Health Service Reorganization: Consultative Document*, London: HMSO.

DHSS (1972) *National Health Service Reorganisation: England*, Cmnd 5055, London: HMSO.

Guillebaud Report (1956) *Report of the Committee of Enquiry into the Cost of the National Health Service*, Cmnd 9663, London: HMSO.

Hodgkinson, R. (1967) *The Origins of the National Health Service: The Medical Services of the New Poor Law 1834–1871*, London: The Wellcome Historical Medical Library.

Klein, R. (1983) *The Politics of the National Health Service*, Harlow: Longman.

Merrison, A. (1979) *Royal Commission on the NHS: Report (Chair: Sir Alec Merrison)*, Cmnd 7615, London: HMSO.

Ministry of Health (1944) *A National Health Service*, Cmd 6502, London: HMSO.

Ministry of Health (1968) *The Administrative Structure of the Medical and Related Services in England and Wales*, First Green Paper, London: HMSO.

Pinker, R. (1966) *English Hospital Statistics 1861–1938*, London: Heinemann.

Pinker, R. (1971) *Social Theory and Social Policy*, London: Heinemann.

Seebohm, F. (1968) *Report of the Committee on Local Authority and Allied Personal Social Services*, Cmnd 3703, London: HMSO.

Thane, P. (1982) *The Foundations of the Welfare State*, Harlow: Longman.

Titmuss, R. M. (1968) *Commitment to Welfare*, London: George Allen & Unwin.

4

Individual Responsiblity or Citizenship Rights?

Ian Kendall and Graham Moon

Introduction

There is an enduring tension between individualist and collectivist conceptions in British health and health care policy. The individualist view fosters notions of individual responsibility for health and (in-dividual) personal choice regarding health care; it is most obviously compatible with the minimal state model of health care and the New Right perspective. In contrast, collectivism embodies ideas of social responsibility and emphasises the importance of social structures and processes in determining and defining health care needs. It is compatible with the universalist/citizenship model of health care and the social democratic perspective. However we should note that other welfare perspectives – feminism, Marxism and welfare plural-ism can also be linked with collectivism since they all include approaches that endorse collective responses, collectivised solutions and state action.

In this chapter, we review the characteristics of individualist and collectivist aspects of health policy before examining the concept of a 'right to health care'. This concept provides a basis for analysing and evaluating different models of state intervention in health care and in particular the New Right perspective. The latter has obvious affinities with long-standing concerns about cost containment in health care, leading perhaps inevitably to the argument that the state should retreat from the universalist/citizenship model to a more selective approach to state involvement in and expenditure on health care. But if the state does less then non-state institutions will have to do more.

67

The focus of this chapter is thus the broad-based concept of the citizen's right to adequate health care rather than the specific entitlements enshrined in the Patient's Charter. For the present it is difficult to see the latter offering any significant extension of health care rights; detailed discussion of the Charter is offered in Chapter 7.

Individualism

The notion of the individualist basis to health policy is central to two usually contradictory but sometimes strangely symbiotic groupings. As suggested above, the policies of privatism and the advocacy of a minimal state model of health care lay a major stress on individualism. This perspective provides a clear underpinning to New Right perspectives which have assumed a much greater political significance in British policies for health and health care since 1979. The second grouping for which notions of individualism are important is the clinicians. For both doctors and nurses, great stress is placed on the provision of care which is individualised, individually focused and tailored to the needs of the individual. There is, of course, an important distinction between these two perspectives. The New Right subscribe to individualism on ideological and political grounds. For the clinicians, the emphasis comes much more from a base in professional ethics. Nevertheless there is an interaction between the perspectives which has served to strengthen an individualist viewpoint. We now explore this interaction.

For the New Right, health problems have individual, atomised explanations. These may be outside the control of the individual, internal to the body, or they may be a consequence of individually chosen autonomous behavioural decisions: lifestyle 'choices' such as smoking, excessive drinking, poor dietary habits, lack of exercise, drug misuse, sexual licence or 'improper' use of health care services. In both cases the solution lies with the individual: an individual decision to use effectively those medical services which are appropriate to the condition, allied to a clear imperative to exercise individual self-reliance and responsibility for one's own actions. Individual needs, individual responsibilities and individualised solutions are core tenets of the New Right perspective. It follows that medicine should treat the individual, not the circumstances which may well underpin health problems, particularly those resulting from 'lifestyle'. This resonates with the training of medical practitioners, which is focused on the treatment of disease in individuals; with 'common sense' insofar as most sick people naturally prefer an individualised intervention to a Utopian equation of their problems with those of society; and with short-term effectiveness, since an individualised medical intervention is preferable to waiting for society to change.

Opposition to this individualised perspective can be problematic. Failure to identify the centrality of the individual as both explanatory unit and potential solution means a fall-back to reliance on the state. For Anderson *et al.* (1983) this brings with it notions of a dependency culture and sheltering from consequences of self-generated problems. As Mohan (1995: 47) puts it: 'Rhetorically, public provision is equated, by some Conservatives, with dependence; private provision, in contrast, is equated with independence and self-reliance.' The promotion of individual responsibility reduces the burden of care carried by the state. In contrast, where individualism is not promoted, the rights of individuals may be stifled by bureaucratic and professional cultures. In essence there is, for the individual, an interplay of rights and obligations in which the individual is both free to act and expected to exercise that freedom (Marshall 1950; Mead, 1985).

Behind this ideological perspective lurks a much more straightforward financial agenda. One of the key pressures facing current governments on a worldwide scale is the escalating costs of providing health care. This cost escalation is bound up in the technological nature of much of current acute medicine and the concomitant drug and equipment costs. This leads to the view that governments cannot afford the costs of modern medicine; the tax or insurance burdens are too onerous to be fiscally sustainable. Consequently the onus for paying for health care is shifted onto the individual consumer. Individualisation is therefore embodied in the continuing health care crisis and, again, simultaneously both an explanation – the crisis is not one of equity or ineffectiveness but one occasioned by the costs of state subsidy – and a solution. In the latter sense, alongside reorganisation and privatisation goes the shift of the direct burden of health care costs onto the individual. The individual is then expected to maximise his or her outcome in the free market where opportunity can be purchased at whatever cost can be sustained by the individual. Navarro (1984), writing on the USA health care system, argues that the New Right claim that too much is spent on the health care bureaucracy and too little on fostering wealth creation. This analysis is equally applicable to the UK and has resulted in the introduction of market elements to correct the perceived inefficiencies of governmental bureaucracy.

A key issue within the New Right framework is the extent to which the individual has the freedom to exercise choice. This matter is particularly stark when considering issues associated with lifestyle and health-related behaviour. As Davison and Davey Smith (1995) argue, one extreme perspective would be that the state has no right to intervene concerning an individual's health-related behaviour: individuals should be free to choose health or illness. Knowles (1977:2) expressed this point succinctly: 'Over 99% of us are born healthy and are made sick as a result of personal misbehaviour . . . the primary critical choice facing the individual is to change his personal habits or stop complaining.' Intervention, in contrast, implies that personal choice is not necessarily right; the (nanny) state may know best.

Governments have tended to develop hybrid approaches to this matter combining a strong commitment to individualisation with a continuing role for the state. *Prevention and Health: everybody's business* (DHSS, 1976a), produced under a British Labour government, states that 'many of the current major problems in prevention are related less to man's outside environment than to his personal behaviour', but prescribed a solution which involved not only the promotion of individual behaviourial change, but also the institutionalisation of surveillance and the use of didactic health education programmes. More recently, the British Conservative government's *The Health of the Nation* (DoH, 1992) promoted similar tactics alongside the promulgation of institutionally determined 'health targets' which fail to allow for individual choice: a paradoxical situation of individual responsibility to conform to institutional norms.

Strong and Robinson (1990) remind us that not only does the impact of individualisation relate to patients/clients and to the explanation and solution through health care of health problems, it also affects the running of a health service. In the UK, the introduction of general management following the Griffiths Report (DHSS, 1983) was, at least conceptually and in part, intended to free those running the NHS from administrative shackles and give them 'freedom' to manage in a more creative and free-wheeling manner. This viewpoint was, of course, rather naive; after Griffiths, people were still looking over their proverbial shoulders. With managerial freedom went managerial accountability and responsibility for action; the managers were freed to manage yet were responsible for their decisions. Rather than fostering individual entrepreneurship and creativity, the result was a lack of strategic vision, responsiveness rather than proactivity, and operationalism rather than innovation. Individuals who did not accept the confines of the role were isolated and a strong corporate identity developed which rather ran counter to ideals of the individualistic manager. Similar processes of exclusion and restructuring were visited upon maverick organisational elements, most notably the Health Education Council, which was converted from a campaigning collectivist body with a chief officer who was highly critical of health policy to, first, an 'authority' with a manager (Beattie 1991) and finally a body dependent upon contract income for its survival.

An attempt to impose an individualised view of health policy on the British NHS ignores the social context of ill-health and the considerable achievements of organised state-led health policy. It also has clear shortcomings as a conceptual, philosophical and theoretical basis for health policy. It assumes that individuals can afford to choose health and buy health care in situations where the state does not provide or purchase. Acceptance of the individualistic approach also legitimises the status quo. Health and health care are atomised and removed from their social context; individuals are exhorted to change and adapt; the structural bases of problems are not addressed. It is arguably this ultimate conservatism which most fundamentally makes the individualist position so central to New Right health policy.

Collectivism

Under a collectivist vision, health policy and its instruments should be collectively owned and/or controlled. The formulation and implementation of policy should not be left to the actions of individuals pursuing their own self-interest. In contrast, both should involve 'higher level' activity with individuals working together in a communitarian or, more usually, statist mode in which the wishes, demands and perhaps even needs of the single individual are secondary to a perceived greater collective benefit. In short, collective or public ownership is expected to deliver greater overall benefits and provide more for the interests of the community as a whole.

Many different forms of social organisation are embodied in this perspective ranging from monolithic state–socialist systems of centralised planning, through varying forms of intervention and regulation, to popular co-operatives. All have, as their hallmark, a commitment to, albeit differing, ideals of organised participation, moderation of the full-blooded impact of markets, social reform and universalism. They claim that markets, on their own, are insufficient to guarantee the rights of individuals; an element of intervention and direction is required to ensure that explanation and solutions are not atomised and that a broader societal perspective is maintained. It might even be claimed that the collectivist notion offers a moral perspective on social order; this idea is, however, rejected by the New Right, who claim a morality for the market (Green, 1990).

In the UK, the collectivist vision of health policy has been most clearly articulated and advanced by 'left of centre' reformist governments – most obviously the pre-First World War Liberal government and post-Second World War Labour governments. Intervening periods of Conservative government have been more contradictory exemplified by the two identifiable strands in New Right perspectives, a considerable sympathy for the 'public burden model of state welfare' (Titmuss, 1968) but a recognition, since 1948, of the enduring popular appeal of the universalist/citizenship model of health care. The outcome for most of the post-war period has been a politically expedient moderation of conflict and a degree of consistency at central government with the direction and strategic shaping of the health care system.

The largely undemocratic local health authorities have been cast in the role of guardians of public interests. The whole basis of the Beveridgian welfare state resonates with collectivist arguments and nowhere are they illustrated more clearly that in the NHS. From the initial nationalisation, through the quest for equality in input most clearly represented by the Resource Allocation Working Party (DHSS 1976b) to the collectivist prescriptions of the Black Report (DHSS 1980), and even on to the ultimately collectivised and paternalistic decision making of the internal market, the collectivity has been a key theme in health policy. Sometimes the guiding force behind this activity has been equality; more recently it has been efficiency (Kendall and Moon, 1990). Generally it has been clear that the manifestation of the collectivity was the state; more recently this clarity has given way to more slippery references to communities and consumer responsiveness (Moon and Brown, 1996). It is not therefore necessarily consistent to see a clear separation of the individual and collective in British health policy and it is certainly incorrect to equate the individual with conservatism and the collective with socialism; *Prevention and Health*, after all, was a Labour document while the concept of health choices promoted by the Conservatives is, if not collective, then at least heavily circumscribed by governmental ideology.

The collectivist critique of individualism is essentially that unfettered individualism breeds inequality and grinds down those who are not in positions of power. Individuals are not in a position to counter these inequalities as they lack resources, power and influence. Supraindividual action is necessary. Collectivist approaches are perhaps most clearly articulated in the Black Report, its diagnosis of a structural basis to health inequality and its prescription of state intervention as the cure. The Black Report went well beyond an individualised approach and sought to 'focus upstream' on the wider causes of health inequality. It found these at the level of social organisation and saw not only health policy but also broader social policies with less obviously direct health effects as a solution. It was decidedly interventionist in tone, arguing for state-led planning and an intersectoral articulation of policy. From a strict collectivist viewpoint it was, of course, irredeemably reformist. It did not challenge the materialist basis of society and saw policy and intervention as a way of ameliorating more deep-seated problems. Yet, more importantly from a realist standpoint, it was dangerously radical to the incoming individualist Conservative government (Carr-Hill, 1987). The subsequent political history of the Black Report is well known and does not bear another repetition. Its rejection, superficially on the grounds of cost, but effectively as a consequence of ideological opposition, has been recounted many times.

Though collectivist approaches using public expenditure need not be a burden but, rather, may be a catalyst for growth – a necessary part of a wise national investment for a thriving economy – it is paradoxically clear from the Black Report's evidence that programmes of state intervention and state guarantees of universal access to health care have been relatively unsuccessful in promoting better health. The World Health Organisation's Healthy Cities approach provides an alternative approach in which, though the state still plays a substantial role, the wider polity is used to construct a broader, potentially more powerful, collectivity stressing the centrality of communities in promoting their own health and participating in otherwise expert-dominated decision-making processes including priority setting (Ashton, 1992, Davies and Kelly, 1993). Target setting, screening, medical care which individualises health problems, and state-led 'top-down' approaches to health care planning are rejected in favour of, or in practice often combined with, notions of empowerment oriented towards real social reform and the promotion of justice and equity (Tesh, 1988).

In a theoretical sense, collectivist approaches are perhaps best seen in relation to debates about citizenship. Though they generally see a role for the state which is considerably greater than that envisaged by the individualist perspective, they need not necessarily imply a statist approach: models of welfare pluralism can be quite compatible with collectivism. The idea of social citizenship with inclusive rights to health care, universal benefits promoting integration into society and obligations to use the services provided need not mean that the state is the provider of the service (Marshall, 1963, 1981). As Plant (1990) has noted, however, individual empowerment is seldom possible without the state; the latter is needed to discriminate in favour of those in greatest need (Pinker, 1988; Titmuss, 1968). Collective empowerment, in contrast, is possible through popular action, through community social movements as well as through the actions of a paternalist state looking after its citizens.

Rights

Running through the two preceding sections of this chapter has been a series of sometimes rather crude dichotomies (Table 4.1). A vertical organisation of these dichotomies illustrates some interesting complementarities in contemporary health policy. At one level these reduce to a dichotomy. On one side better health is attained through looking holistically at health problems, responding collectively, involving the state and focusing on the production of ill-health. On the other side there is a concentration on the individualised needs of the sick person and satisfying those needs in ways that can be specifically aimed at

TABLE 4.1   *The collective and the individual:*
dichotomies and resonances

Collective	Individual
social	medical
state	market
public	private
holistic	atomised
universal	specific
left	right

individual problems rather than addressed through generalised, non-specific strategies. On another level, it is also possible to explore the themes of collectivism and individualism in health policy in relation to rights to health care. It is to this task that we now turn.

Both individual and collective rights have a long history in British health policy. The emerging Poor Law medical service meant that 'the poor had gained the right to institutional care when they were sick' (Abel-Smith, 1964: 65). The consequent duty of the state to provide hospitals for the poor received its first formal acknowledgement in the Metropolitan Poor Act of 1867 (Ayers, 1971: 1). Further rights to health care were embodied in the National Health Insurance Act 1911 through the associated obligation to pay National Insurance contributions. However such rights were not universal but limited to contributors (see Chapter 3). The subsequent establishment of the NHS can be seen to represent a much more profound commitment to individual rights guaranteed by the state. All citizens were entitled to use a state funded, comprehensive health service which was largely free of service-user charges and for which entitlements were not limited by social and economic circumstances but were a genuine badge of citizenship. However, as indicated by the differing perspectives identified in Chapter 1, the concept of a citizenship right to welfare, including a right to health care, has remained an area of controversy and conflict.

The position of some radical right writers that 'medical care would appear to have no characteristics which differentiate it sharply from other goods in the market' (Lees, 1965: 39) seems to conflict with any state intervention in health care at all – even that associated with the minimal state model of health care available through the nineteenth-century Poor Law authorities. It is certainly at odds with social democratic perspectives that emphasise the problems of market-based allocations of health care (Titmuss, 1968: 146–7). In reality few critics of the universalist/citizenship model of health care advocate the total abandonment of state responsibilities for health care.

This seems to follow from what may have been a grudging acceptance of a right to minimal health care. Of course the concept of a right to minimal health care does not lead immediately to some sort of state intervention: it might be realised through alternative providers and alternative forms of funding. The New Right have always argued the virtues of such alternatives to state welfare (see Chapter 1), these being (a) profit and competition – health care through the market and employers; (b) altruism and mutual aid – health care through voluntary associations; and (c) informal caring networks – health care through families and communities.

With regard to profit and competition, the major mechanism is private insurance, since few individuals can afford to pay on demand when medical need arises. The potential for such private insurance in the area of health care is considerable (as the example of the USA indicates). The operation of such a market/private insurance based system of health care has traditionally raised a number of concerns relating to both inequalities and inefficiencies. However, while we may have justifiable concerns about the extent to which markets in health care do not match up to the benefits (choice and efficiency) of the theoretical model, a more fundamental issue concerns groups whom the insurance industry will effectively label as the 'bad risks of an industrial economy'. For these 'bad risks', the limitations of health care markets will be of less concern than their inability to enter the market in the first place. The classic 'bad risks' for health care insurance may include elderly people, people with physical disabilities and people with chronic health problems.

Employer-based welfare schemes may include health care, and extend the market beyond those who can afford conventional health insurance provision, but the evidence on deregulated occupational welfare suggests a pattern of inequalities and exclusions that replicate that of market and insurance-based provision. Most obviously serious health problems can lead to a marginal position in, or exclusion from, the labour market and the latter is inevitably associated with little or no access to occupational welfare.

Philanthropic and mutual aid voluntary associations have played a key role in the development of health care in most industrial societies, as we noted in Chapter 3. In Europe, contemporary health care systems are invariably based upon the foundations of charitable hospitals and medical benefits provided by mutual aid organisations (trade unions and Friendly Societies). However this historical role also provides ample evidence of the potential limitations of a reliance on altruism and mutual aid as the means of providing a right to minimal health care (see Chapter 3). Despite their considerable merits as providers of good-quality hospital care to those who would be unable to purchase such care in a private market, Britain's voluntary hospitals were limited in their coverage both to certain areas of the country and to certain areas of health care. The mutual aid institutions of nineteenth century Britain – the Friendly Societies – were also limited in their coverage of the population. Whether a modern day version of mutual aid would be more successful is equally questionable; contemporary health care examples indicate that non-profit voluntary health insurance institutions, like Blue Cross in the USA, have to adjust their premiums to risks or they will be left with the bad risks, as the good risks are offered cheaper policies elsewhere (Abel-Smith, 1976).

For the New Right, families and communities constitute another set of alternative welfare institutions who might reasonably reclaim their historical role as pre-eminent welfare institutions and thus aid the replacement of extensive state welfare activity. This perspective seems to be at least in part based on assumptions that the family and state are competing welfare institutions and that the diminished contemporary welfare role for families is attributable to an extending and intrusive role for the state. Diminish the role of its competitor by 'rolling back the frontiers of the welfare state' and the frontiers of the 'welfare family' are presumed to begin expanding. This perspective conflicts most obviously with traditional sociological perspectives which agree with the trend but reverse the causal relationship. The changes in the family have been caused by fundamental changes in structure and function brought about by industrialisation and urbanisation and the changing role for families becomes one of the factors leading to an increased health and welfare role for the state, rather than the other way round. From this perspective you would need to 'roll back the frontiers of industrialisation and urbanisation' before you diminished the welfare role of the state – unless you were indifferent to significant social and economic consequences of poverty and deprivation.

Another perspective on the family and the state maintains that the so-called dramatic 'decline' in the welfare role of families and communities has been overstated. At one end of the time continuum, historians have questioned the historical veracity of extended families as effective welfare institutions and, at the other end, social policy researchers have undertaken a more precise delineation of a formidable army of contemporary informal carers. On this reading there is no necessary contradiction or competition between state welfare and familial welfare: the former may support the latter and to diminish the state's role might actually diminish the ability of informal carers to sustain their major role in health and social care. There are also questions about the ability and desirability of substituting familial care for the sort of specialised nursing and other forms of care and support that could be delivered through a state health care system like the NHS. Reliance on families also raises concerns about inequalities in familial resources: compare a large, rich family with an impoverished single-parent family with few relations and consider that some people have little or no kin.

These widely recognised limitations of non-state providers of health care lead critics of state intervention, not to an advocacy of the NHS, but rather to an acceptance of a modern day version of the Poor Law – the minimal state model of health care. This will provide a safety net for those whose health care needs remain unmet by the markets, communities, associations and altruism. Continuing concerns relating to costs and cost containment also provide the basis for a return to the minimal state model of health care on the grounds that the state cannot afford the public expenditures associated with the universalist/ citizenship model. Indeed this criticism has been directed at the NHS virtually since its inception. Concerns relating to the financial implications of demographic trends for the costs of state welfare and the redistribution of wealth endangering 'the social well-being of the nation' were well-established features of political debate in the early 1950s (Phillips, 1954; Conservative Political Centre, 1950). One seemingly attractive proposition is that limited government resources should be concentrated on those individuals in greatest need. Individualised direction of services to the least well off provides the opportunity to deliver civilised living standards for all, with less burdensome taxation. Needless to say, this is not a new idea (see MacLeod and Powell, 1949: 4) and the debate between the universalism (exemplified by the National Health Service) and more individualised or 'selective' approaches (exemplified by Income Support and Family Credit) has a long history. Since the selective approach has obvious superficial attractions, it is perhaps most helpful to remind ourselves of some of the associated problems and dilemmas.

Although invariably involving less public expenditure overall, a selective approach incurs high administrative costs – perhaps an inevitable consequence of the complexity of schemes that seek to aim a service at a limited section of the population and to exclude the rest of the population. There are clearly issues of equity associated with this complexity, most obviously ensuring that services *are not received* by people who are 'not really poor' and *are received* by those in greatest need.

Another consistently and widely reported problem of selectivity is that of underutilisation: not all those members of the community at which the services are directed come forward to claim them. This may reflect a number of factors, including a stigma attributed to means testing and the difficulties of understanding the complexities of entitlement. Of course the understanding of potential service-users, and those who advise them, may be resolved by simplifying rules of entitlement, but simpler rules may entail a degree of 'rough justice' that denies benefits to some while conferring benefits on others in a manner that offends the community's sense of 'natural justice'. A 'rough justice' approach is likely to lead to a situation where services *are not received* by people who 'really need them', and *are received* by those who are 'less deserving'.

The fundamental dilemma of more selective approaches lies in their apparent inability to deliver good-quality services to the neediest members of a society. If this promise could be fulfilled, more expensive universalist services could be abandoned; and it is hoped that improved organisation, information and advice would resolve the problems of administrative costs, equity and underutilisation. But a central criticism of selectivity relates to the concern that a 'health service for the poor is likely to be a poor health service'.

This leads to a key question of whether selectivity is inevitably associated with poor-quality services and stigma. This is partly an empirical question. But it is also possible to locate these problems as inextricably bound up with the principles underpinning the selective approach. For example, providing a poor quality service may deter potential users and ameliorate the problem of excluding those considered to be 'less needy' – an approach most obviously associated with the 'workhouse test' of the New Poor Law (see Chapter 3).

The market situation of selective state services may also contribute to poor quality. As they seek to compete for resources, especially staff, against major private sector institutions, they may end up with the worst rather than the best professionals and managers. This disadvantaged market situation may be exacerbated by the political situation. The wholesale adoption of selectivity would seem to imply a broad acceptance by the community of an approach which makes a necessary virtue out of restraining and restricting all forms of public expenditure on social services (the 'public burden' model of state welfare). This is likely to influence the scale and scope of expenditure on selective services, with a consequent impact on the quality of those services. Most pertinently it seems unlikely that the majority of the electorate, by definition excluded from access to services aimed at a needy minority, will seek to increase taxes on themselves to provide good quality services for that minority. This is especially true of those in the income range just excluded by selective provision who will be struggling with the impact of health insurance premiums, private pension contributions and school fees on their own household budgets. If market and political forces lead to selective services which are of poor quality, those services will certainly not enhance the status of those that use them. Furthermore a concern with the 'burden of taxation' will define expenditure on selective social services as a 'public burden' and consign those who use those services to a similar, devalued and stigmatised category.

A final criticism of selectivity relates to the problem of disincentives associated with the extensive systems of means testing. Even in the British situation where the social security system retains some universalist cash benefits (for example, child benefit) and operates in a context of universal health and education systems, researchers have consistently documented the extent to which a substantial body of low-wage earners may be subjected to the powerful disincentive effects of interlocking means-tested benefits. This brings us to a particular problem of selectivity, at least for those who claim that it affords the opportunity to aim better benefits at the disadvantaged and so redistribute resources more effectively. Problems of disincentives, and indeed concerns about abuse, costs, equity and knowledge, may all be minimised or resolved by providing simple to understand and obviously poor-quality services – basically by reinventing some sort of modern-day version of the mid-nineteenth century Poor Law (see Chapter 3).

It is when we seek to use selectivity as a device for delivering good-quality services to the poorest members of society that the dilemmas and problems arise. For the critics of universalist 'welfare state programmes', often much concerned with questions of 'economic efficiency' and 'dependency cultures', there is a real dilemma. It is to the extension of state welfare that a variety of economic and social ills have been attributed, notably expensive universalist provision. But it is selectivity, not universalism, that poses the significant problems for the operation of sizeable sections of the labour market, creating a 'dependency culture' where many individuals, families and households are locked into economic circumstances where rises in income and/or savings disqualify them from access to means-tested benefits and services. To 'roll back the frontiers of the welfare state' so that access to education, health care and pensions was also means-tested would be to further compound this problem. Only a form of selectivity that effectively and systematically penalises all disadvantaged and poor people, rather than just the disreputable members of the 'underclass', can avoid this problem of disincentives and 'poverty traps'.

Despite its superficial attractions it seems likely that a modern state welfare system constructed entirely around the principle of selectivity will consign significant minorities within society to levels of education, health care and pensions that the majority of the population would regard as quite unacceptable for themselves and their families. Thus a move to selectivity can contribute to an overall reduction in public expenditure and hence in the 'burden of taxation'. What it is unlikely to achieve is the provision of reasonable quality services to the most needy. Furthermore, if this theoretical possibility was made reality, there would be a most profound problem of disincentives to work and save. To seek to provide decent services for disadvantaged groups through selectivity would seem to be ideologically inconsistent, socially undesirable, economically problematic and politically impossible.

Conclusions

Individualist and collectivist conceptions of health and health care can provide the rationales for radically different policy agendas. In the end the continuum of policy options is narrowed somewhat by the widespread consensus around, on the one hand, the notion that the state should assume responsibility for guaranteeing some minimal rights to minimal health care and, on the other, the idea that the health status of communities, groups and individuals will often owe something to individual choices. Nonetheless this still leaves considerable scope for major differences of opinion about the role of the state in matters of health and health care. In the end a crucial value conflict concerns the right to adequate health care. If a community adopts the principle that all members of that community should have a reasonable expectation that their needs for a reasonable standard of health care will be met, there is compelling evidence to say that such a community should have something like a National Health Service.

Bibliography

Abel-Smith, B. (1964) *The Hospitals 1800–1948 : a study in social administration in England and Wales*, London: Heinemann.

Abel-Smith, B. (1976) *Value for Money in Health Services*, London: Heinemann.

Anderson, D., Lait, J. and Marsland, D. (1983) *Breaking the Spell of the Welfare State*, London: Centre for Policy Studies.

Ashton, J. (1992) *Healthy Cities*, Buckingham: Open University Press.

Ayers, G. (1971) *England's First State Hospitals and the Metropolitan Asylums Board 1867–1930*, London: Wellcome Institute of the History of Medicine.

Beattie, A. (1991) 'Knowledge and control in health promotion: a test case for social policy and social theory', in J. Gabe, M. Calnan and M. Bury (eds) , *The Sociology of the Health Service*, London: Routledge.

Bunton, R. *et al.* (eds) (1995) *The Sociology of Health Promotion: critical analyses of consumption, lifestyle and risk*, London: Routledge.

Carr-Hill, R. (1987) 'The inequalities in health debate: a critical review of the issues', in R. Bunton, S. Nettleton and R. Burrows, *Journal of Social Policy*, vol. 16, pp. 509–42.

Conservative Political Centre (1950) *One Nation*, London: Conservative Political Centre.

Davies, J. and Kelly, M. (1993) *Healthy Cities*, London: Routledge.

Davison, C. and Davey Smith, G. (1995) 'The baby and the bath water: examining socio-cultural and free-market critiques of health promotion', in R. Bunton, *et al.* (eds) *The Sociology of Health Promotion*, London: Routledge.

DHSS (1976a) *Prevention and Health: everybody's business*, London: DHSS.

DHSS (1976b) *Sharing Resources for Health in England*, London: DHSS.

DHSS (1980) *Inequalities in Health*, Report of a Research Working Group chaired by Sir Douglas Black, London: DHSS.

DHSS (1983) *NHS Management Inquiry Report*, London: HMSO.

DoH (1992) *The Health of the Nation*, Cmnd 1523, London: HMSO.

Gabe, J., Calnan, M. and Bury, M. (eds) (1991) *The Sociology of the Health Service*, London: Routledge.

Green, D. (1990) *Equalising People*, IEA Health and Welfare Unit, Choices in Welfare Series No. 4., London: IEA Health and Welfare Unit.

Green, D. (ed.) (1988) *Acceptable Inequalities: essays on the pursuit of equality in health care*, London: IEA Health Unit Paper No. 3, IEA Health Unit.

Ham, C., Robinson, R. and Benzeval, M. (1990) *Health Check*, London: Kings Fund Institute.

Harris, R. (ed.) (1965) *Freedom or Free for All? Essays in welfare, trade and choice*, London: Institute of Economic Affairs.

Kearns, R. and Gesler, W. (eds) (1996).

Kendall, I. and Moon, G. (1990) 'Health policy' in S. Savage and L. Robins (eds) (1990).

Knowles, J. (1977) *Doing Better, Feeling Worse: health in the United States*, New York: Norton Press.

Lees, D. (1965) 'Health Through Choice' in R. Harris (ed.), *Freedom or Free for All?*, London: Institute of Economic Affairs.

MacLeod, I. and Powell, E. (1949) *The Social Services – Needs and Means*, London: Conservative Political Centre.

Marshall, T. (1950) *Citizenship and Social Class*, Cambridge: CUP.

Marshall, T. (1963) *Sociology at the Crossroads and Other Essays*, London: Heinemann.

Marshall, T. (1981) *The Right to Welfare and Other Essays*, London: Heinemann.

Mead, L. (1985) *Beyond Entitlement*, New York: Basic Books.

Mohan, J. (1995) *A National Health Service*, Basingstoke: Macmillan.

Moon, G. and Brown, T. (1996) 'Place, space and the reform of the British National Health Service' in R. Kearns and W. Gesler (eds), *Putting Health into Place: landscape identity and wellbeing*, Syracuse, NY: Syracuse University Press.

Navarro, V. (1984) 'Selected myths guiding the Reagan administration's health policies', *International Journal of Health Services*, vol. 13, pp. 179–202.

Phillips Report (1954) *Report of the Committee on the Economic and Financial Problems of the Provision for Old Age*, Cmd 9333, London: HMSO.

Pinker, R. (1988) 'Towards a mixed economy of welfare in health care' in D. Green (ed.), *Acceptable Inequalities*, London: IEA Health Unit.

Plant, R. (1990) 'Citizenship and Rights', in *Citizenship and Rights in Thatcher's Britain: two views*, IEA Health and Welfare Unit, Choices in Welfare Series No. 3, London: IEA Health and Welfare Unit, pp. 1–32.

Savage, S. and Robins, L. (eds) (1990) *Public Policy under Thatcher*, London: Macmillan.

Strong, P. and Robinson, J. (1990) *The NHS – under new management*, Buckingham: Open University Press.

Tesh, S. (1988) *Hidden Arguments: political ideology and disease prevention policy*, New Brunswick, NJ: Rutgers University Press.

Titmuss, R. M. (1968) *Commitment to Welfare* (1968) London: George Allen & Unwin.

Townsend, P. and Davidson, N. (1982) *Inequalities in Health*, Harmondsworth: Penguin.

5

Managers and Professionals

Rosemary Gillespie

Introduction

Previous chapters have explored the ways in which a period of industrial and social development led to the development of welfare states, and in particular health policies and services in a welfare context. This period of social development, or 'modernity', also witnessed the emergence of powerful occupational groups that came to be known as the 'professions'. The transformations of nineteenth-century British society due to the development of industrial capitalism led to considerable upheaval in social structure. This resulted in what Perkin has termed 'professional society' (1989:2), whereby certain occupational groups were able to privilege themselves over other workers and achieve power, prestige and high economic reward. This chapter will first examine the meaning and significance of the professions, in particular the professions involved in the delivery of health care. A range of traditional and critical approaches to the professions and professional power will be examined. Second, the rise of professional power in the delivery of health care will be explored by reviewing the influential position of the medical profession since 1948. The chapter will provide an overview of the changes to the service that have had an impact on professional power following the implementation of the recommendations of the Griffiths Report. In particular it will review the emergence of general management in the NHS and evaluate the extent to which the radicalism of the 'new managerialism' (Davidson, 1987) has successfully contested medical hegemony. Conflicts, allegiances and changes in the balance

84

of power will be examined in the light of health service reforms in the 1990s as well as the implications of these for patients, nurses and other paramedical groups.

Professionals and Professional Power

Since the Industrial Revolution, and the development of capitalism and industrialisation in Britain, considerable changes to the occupational structure of society have emerged. Capitalist entrepreneurs have comprised one powerful and affluent group following these changes, but this era has also precipitated the rapid establishment and growth of other powerful occupational groups, the professions. With the onset of industrialisation the professions mushroomed and their client base, drawn from the new bourgeoisie, expanded (Perkin, 1989). They have come to hold a high status and command high financial rewards because much of modern social life involves knowledge, expertise and the transmission of specialist information (Giddens, 1989). The medical profession is an example of an occupational group that has achieved this power and influence *par excellence*. Medicine, with its armoury of techniques, technologies and drugs, has undertaken to treat and cure disease, relieve suffering and improve both quality and length of life, and has generally been seen to act in the interests of individuals and society. Furthermore, in an increasingly secular society, medical power has, in many ways, come to replace that of ecclesiastical regulation. Turner (1987), for example, has argued that the human body has become an object of science rather than a focus of theology. Medical classifications of deviance have largely replaced confessional practice, while sin has been replaced by science, medicine increasingly determines appropriate and inappropriate behaviour (Zola, 1972). The profession of medicine can therefore be seen to regulate human social life in highly significant ways.

Professionals may work in the private sector as individuals or in groups or firms, for example the legal profession, and are often in a position to secure virtual monopolistic fees. Professionals may also be employed in the public sector. The social reforms of the nineteenth century and the collectivist ideology of the early twentieth century gave rise to a proliferation of professional groups in areas such as preventive medicine, sanitary engineering and central and local government. Thus the patron or customer became the entire community and much professional expertise came to be underwritten by the state (Perkin, 1989). Since the beginning of the welfare state, a prime example of this has been the medical profession in the National Health Service (NHS). When employed in large organisations, professionals command a greater degree of autonomy over their role than others, and are able to stand apart from a bureaucratic framework. Doctors in the NHS, for example, are able to do this in ways that other workers within an organisational hierarchy cannot.

Traditional Approaches to the Professions

Traditional explanatory approaches to the sociology of the professions conceptualised that professionals, for example the legal profession, the clergy and the medical profession, can be distinguished from other social groups by their sense of personal service to others and 'altruism', rather than the desire for economic reward; that they are 'collectively oriented' rather than 'self-oriented' (Johnson, 1972; Turner, 1987). One dominant and influential explanatory framework in relation to the professions has been that of the 'trait approach' (Millerson, 1964; Greenwood, 1957). This approach highlights the existence of certain traits or characteristics that professionals have in common that mark them off from the rest of society. Traits of the professions include theoretical knowledge as a basis of competence; the development of freedom and self-governance over their education and training; formal examinations, whereby the more complex the knowledge base and the more inaccessible it is to lay people, the more likely is a group able to demand professional status; a professional organisation; a code of conduct; and finally, altruism. The knowledge is thus seen to be used for the public good, giving rise to trust (Millerson, 1964).

A further explanatory account of the professions is that of Parsons (1954). Parsons' functionalist account espoused the belief that professional groups constitute a stabilising force in capitalist society, working for the common good. This was seen to counter the dominant ethos of capitalism, which is principally the pursuit of profit (Turner, 1987). The functionalist approach explains the high social standing traditionally enjoyed by members of a profession on the basis of the services they offer and their high levels of knowledge, resulting in the esteem in which society holds them and the maintenance of a stable social system. Traditional approaches, therefore, define professions in terms of particular qualities and the benefits they provide to society as a whole.

Critical Approaches to the Professions

Traditional explanatory theories of the professions such as the trait and functionalist approaches have been criticised for their largely uncritical analysis. First, definitions of what constitutes a profession are based on the profession's own account, that of the elite groups themselves. Second, these analyses ignore the power, privilege and social position held by professional groups that may be seen to serve their own interests, rather than those of society (Turner, 1987). Critical accounts, developed in the 1970s and 1980s, principally concerned with the notion of power, have questioned the benefits for society of the services provided by the professions, highlighting the monopolistic practices and self-interests that may be served by such groups. Hugman (1991) has argued that traits should themselves be subject to investigation rather than simply be accepted as 'fact'. Johnson has highlighted the ways professions have presented a 'Janus-head' (1972: 17). On the one hand, they may be seen to provide a buffer from a world of bureaucracy and market forces, yet they themselves may provide a threat to society through their own monopolistic practices and self-interest.

Marxist critiques of professional power have provided an analysis that draws on class divisions. Johnson (1972, 1977, 1982), for example, suggests that, in studying the professions, two fundamental questions are raised (1972: 10). First, are the professions a product of the division of labour? Does, for example, industrialised society create the need for groups that are set apart from other workers? Or second, do they perform a unique social function in industrialised society, which may be economic, political or social? Johnson examines professions in terms of the development of power structures. He argues that there are three types of professional structure: first, the collegiate profession, whereby power is exerted by members of the profession through the emergence of an autonomous occupational association, for example the emergence of the Royal Colleges and the British Medical Association. Second, in the patronage model, power is exercised between professionals and those who pay for services. The consumer defines her/his own needs and the manner in which they will be met, for example private medicine, and increasingly dental care, in the UK in the 1990s. Third, Johnson defines a mediated profession, whereby power is mediated between producer and consumer through a third party who may define both the needs and the ways in which they are met. An example of this may be the ways in which the state mediates medical services within the National Health Service.

The Marxist critique of the professions also explores the privileged position that members of professions hold in the labour market and their links with capital accumulation. Navarro (1976) and Doyal (1979) have been critical of the direct role of medicine in capital accumulation. This is seen both in the private market that exists in medical care and in the market created for equipment and drugs. Navarro in particular has been critical of the dominance of the medical model and has emphasised the relationship between capitalist production and ill health. Other writers drawing on a Marxist analysis such as Oppenheimer (1973) and McKinlay and Arches, (1985), have drawn on a theory of proletarianisation, or loss of professional dominance, to explain what they describe as a transformation of labour processes that medicine has begun to undergo. This transformation, proletarianisation theorists argue, involves a progressive loss of skills and autonomy, and subsequently a loss of power and dominance on the part of the professionals. This loss is manifest in the deskilling and the fragmentation of knowledge caused by increased specialisation, and greater use of technology in medicine. In addition, loss of control over decision making arises through, for example, managerial control and challenges from an increasingly informed lay public. The effect of this is for doctors to lose much of their power as their social and cultural supremacy is challenged (Elston, 1991). Much of the literature about proletarianisation refers to the American health care system, but some of these processes are increasingly evident in the rapidly changing NHS of the 1990s.

A further challenge to traditional approaches to the sociology of the professions is the neo-Weberian critique. Weber perceived the social world to be made up of groups and group interests, with certain groups securing the ability to dominate others. Within this position professions are themselves dominated by, and linked to, the monopolistic interests and bureaucratic forces of capitalism (Turner, 1987). The neo-Weberian concept of exclusionary closure illustrates how the exclusion of others enables a group to control the number of entrants

(Parry and Parry, 1976; Parkin, 1979). A profession, therefore, through exclusionary closure maintains its exclusivity and protects its high economic rewards. Freidson (1970), writing primarily about the American health care system, was critical of the medical profession for their monopolistic and dominating practice in the provision of health services. He contested the entrenched power of the profession, its dominant position in the division of labour and its ability to subordinate other groups of workers. He argued that, rather than altruism, the profession is motivated by its own interests and privileges. Freidson's approach stresses that, instead of acting as a buffer from the world of capitalism and market forces, professional groups are contained within, and are part of, the capitalist economy. Rather than rising above self-interest, professional groups are themselves immersed in the production of wealth, through high fees for their services. The wider the social distance between client and professional, and the greater the helplessness of the client, the greater the exposure to possible exploitation and therefore the need for regulation and control (Johnson, 1972). In a medical encounter, this type of social distance is seen when doctors adopt what Parsons (1951) has termed the 'paternalistic', clinical practice style.

A further critique of the professions is that provided by feminists. This focuses on both the gendered division of labour within professional groups and the treatment of women by professional groups. First, occupations that have successfully achieved professional status, in terms of dominance and autonomy, have principally been male occupations (Stacey, 1988). Female occupations have prospered less well in the organisational hierarchy, in groups termed by Etzioni (1969) 'semi-professions', for example nurses, midwives and social workers. Witz (1992) has developed a theory of patriarchy and professions which has drawn on the neo-Weberian concept of closure. In her gendered analysis of power in occupational groups, she argues that patriarchal relations in nineteenth-century culture excluded women from higher education and therefore from influence in the public sphere. This virtual exclusion of women significantly influenced the nature of the development of professional organisations, enabling them to achieve a male professional profile and subsequently gendered occupational closure (Witz, 1992; Glazer and Slater, 1987).

Crompton (1987) has argued that closure occurs at the individual or micro societal level through interactions between individual men and women in the workplace, such as sexual harassment. It also works, she contends, at the macro societal or collective level, whereby groups of male workers seek to exclude, or deny entry to women through strategies such as 'Old Boys' Networks', and denial of women's suitability for certain roles. One example includes resistance to the entry of women to key roles in the armed forces. Witz has highlighted how, in relation to gender, closure is both exclusionary (Parkin, 1979) and demarcationary (Kreckel, 1980). Exclusionary closure involves the exercising of power downwards as a means of subordinating other occupational groups in order to maintain or enhance power, rewards or privilege (Witz, 1992). Demarcation, or the segregation of women into particular, separate, occupations, is a further means of controlling and regulating occupational groups. The medical profession, the dental profession and the legal profession constitute examples of groups deploying both exclusionary and demarcationary closure in their dealings with allied occupational groups. In all these examples the key professional occupation is dominated by men, yet is supported by several female dominated, subordinate 'semi-professional' occupational groups, such as nurses, hygienists, secretaries, clerks and receptionists.

Feminism has also highlighted the ways in which the medical profession is of historical and primary significance in determining women's unequal social position (Ehrenreich and English, 1979; Bleir, 1988; Stacey, 1988; Oakley, 1993; Martin, 1989). This is evident at both the individual level, through face-to-face encounters with doctors (Foster, 1989), and the social level, through medical endorsement of patriarchal ideology (Martin, 1989). The power of the medical profession over women's embodiment is evident through the medicalisation of, and control over, female sexuality, fertility, contraception, reproduction and mental health. As a result women's bodies have become a primary site for medicalisation and oppression (Oakley, 1984, 1993; Savage, 1986; Miles, 1988; Ussher, 1991). Kohler Reissman (1989) has shown how the continued and increased medicalisation of women's problems, such as infertility, endometrio-sis, menopause and premenstrual syndrome, has functioned both in the interests of physicians who define illness and monopolise treat-ment and in the interests of women who have collaborated in medicalisation to further their own needs and class-specific interests. Finally feminist writers like Scully and Bart (1978) and Moore and Clarke (1995) have explored the ways women are marginalised and denigrated by the medical profession through the ways they are depicted in gynaecology and anatomy textbooks.

The medicalisation of human social life has been criticised by writers who have argued that medicine has served to create the need for its services by medicalising the commonplace problems associated with human life (Zola, 1972). Similarly Illich (1976), although writing from a philosophical libertarian perspective, has presented an argument that has subsequently been developed further by the New Right. Illich argued that reliance on experts such as doctors is pathological for society and individuals. He suggests that the medical establishment has become a major threat to health through the disabling impact of professional control, creating an 'iatrogenic pandemic' (1976). Iatrogenesis, the production of pain, sickness and death as a result of medical care, occurs, Illich argues, at three levels: first, clinical iatrogenesis, which is seen to be the pain dysfunction and disability that results from medical intervention; second, social iatrogenesis, whereby the expansion of medicine creates an artificial and ever expanding market for its services; third, structural iatrogenesis, that undermines people's competence in caring for and confronting death.

The New Right, furthering the individualistic position put forward by Illich, has adopted an approach that has attacked the ways in which the medical profession has maintained a powerful grip on services and resources in health care. The health policies of Thatcherism and Majorism in the UK in the 1980s and 1990s have been influenced by the ideologies of political liberalism, monetarism and free market economics that have advocated a smaller role for the state in economic and social affairs. Such an ethos represents a considerable change from the socialist and consensus philosophies within which the NHS was established (Cox, 1992). It has brought about a desire to deregulate and challenge the power of the trade unions and the professions, including medicine and dentistry, and impose controls on public spending. It has also led to the introduction into health care of commercial practices and the discipline of the market (ibid.). New Right philosophy sees freedom as being threatened by the power that bureaucrats and professionals hold. Professional dominance and hegemony over health care have been challenged by the introduction of radical reforms in relation to management, funding, community care, primary care and public health. The effects of these reforms will be explored further in the final section of this chapter.

Finally medical hegemony has also been challenged as a by-product of a process of wider social change. This has become evident in two areas of health care delivery: first, the increased use of alternative, complementary and self-help therapies, and second, the emergence of an increasingly knowledgeable and assertive consumer of medical services. Saks (1994) has highlighted that as many as one in seven of the population attend alternative practitioner services for treatments such as acupuncture, osteopathy, homeopathy and, more recently, aromatherapy, reflexology and crystal therapy. In alternative therapies patients also adopt a system of self-referral which undermines the tradition of medical referral. This trend, which may indicate a growing dissatisfaction with traditional medicine, has become particularly significant over the last couple of decades.

The second area of social change, increased assertiveness by the consumers of services, may have been brought about, at least in part, by government policy through the Patient's Charter, which forms part of the Conservative government's Citizen's Charter published in 1992. The Charter sets out a range of rights and promises in relation to patient care. It has challenged professional dominance in many parts of the service by increasing patients' expectations and detailing a procedure by which they may make a complaint. This movement may also be linked to the trend of increasing litigation for medical negligence (Dingwall, 1994).

Traditional approaches to the professions have come under attack from a range of theoretical and policy perspectives. Such challenges to professional dominance increasingly undermine the high status of professional groups. The medical profession, in particular, has been criticised at both micro and macro-societal levels, by the left, the right and feminism, and through process, as associated with wider social change. Challenges to medical power through New Right-influenced government policy and the rise of the professional manager will be examined in the following section.

The Rise of Professional Power in Health Care

The profession of medicine gained in strength and prestige as it became the arbitrator of the provision of medical services both within nationalised services of the NHS and in the private sector. Harrison and Pollitt argue that, in particular in the NHS, the shape of the service was an 'aggregate outcome of individual doctors' clinical decisions, rather than the result of decisions made by politicians, policy makers, planners or managers' (1994: 35).

However the history of the profession, far from being that of a homogeneous group, is itself fraught with conflicts and divisions, in particular between GPs, largely represented by the British Medical Association (BMA) and hospital consultants represented by the Royal Colleges (Stacey, 1988). Discord has also arisen between hospital consultants of different specialities as they fight for increasingly scarce resources. Fox (1992), in his sociological analysis of the sphere of the operating theatre, has highlighted the conflict, and at times antagonism, that can arise between surgeons and anaesthetists as a consequence of their different roles and distinct discourses. Similarly in the late 1980s junior hospital doctors, in their demands for a shorter working week, opposed, for the first time, some of their senior colleagues. This resulted in the publication of *The New Deal* (DoH, 1991), announcing intentions to limit the hours junior doctors worked. Doctors, it appears, are like football supporters, who extend tribal loyalty to their local team on Saturdays, and yet in the wider arena can all be seen to support the national team.

The emergence of an affluent professional medical elite in Britain in the nineteenth and twentieth centuries resulted in a new status for those within it. Nursing, however, as Stacey (1988) and Witz (1992) have highlighted, had a significantly different history. Caring for the sick had generally taken place in the domestic sphere, with those paid to perform caring duties counted amongst domestic servants. Gradually the work of nurses was removed from the household into the hospital, with the emergence of what Jewson (1976) has termed 'hospital medicine', with nursing activities principally supportive of medicine. Early in the twentieth century the Nurse Registration Act (1919) was passed. Following a long struggle by key figures within nursing, the 'profession' had become formalised and subject to training and regulation. However regulation was largely by the medical profession, to which nurses remained subordinate (Stacey, 1988; Witz, 1992). Although nurses comprised one of the three occupational hierarchies in the NHS, medicine, nursing and administration, nurses predominantly executed instructions given by doctors in the care of patients (Stacey, 1988). The Salmon Report in

1966 established a new hierarchy within nursing and gave it a role, albeit limited, in health management. Despite this, however, nursing remained subordinate to medicine and its role in policy making remained limited.

Similarly, under the Midwives Act (1902), after 1910 only certified midwives, who held a recognised qualification in midwifery, regulated by the medical profession, could 'habitually and for gain' attend women in labour (Leap and Hunter, 1993: 4–6). Thus working class handywomen, who had cared for women in labour for generations, were virtually excluded from the formal provision of midwifery services. Qualified midwives who provided care did so under the supervision of medical men (ibid.).

In response to changing society and different health challenges, many of the 'semi-professions' have attempted to increase their professional position through graduate status and attempting to increase autonomy over their occupational practice, as with radiography and physiotherapy. Nursing has also launched an education revolution in recent years with the development of a new, more academic programme of learning. Through the 'new nursing' (Davis, 1995) nurses are attempting to fulfil the criteria for professional status. For example, they have a professional body, a code of conduct and, more recently, a period of study in higher education. Nevertheless, of all health professionals, doctors have been able to maintain the principal influence over health policy.

Medical Influence on Health Policy Since 1948

Through their influential and privileged social position, doctors have been seen to be powerful social players in ways that have enabled them to influence the organisational culture and ethos of the National Health Service since its inception in 1948.

Prior to the creation of the service there had been fierce opposition to a national service by the BMA, who indignantly resented greater state control over their services (Klein, 1989). The strong bargaining position of doctors enabled them to negotiate their demands, in the light of fears that doctors would not co-operate with the new service. For example, a memorandum from Sir Arthur MacNalty, the Chief Medical Officer to the Ministry of Health, in September 1939, stated that there was a need for 'a National Health Service established by negotiation with the general agreement of the medical profession' (quoted in Klein, 1989: 8).

Doctors were able to insist that their views should be represented despite a statement in a White Paper (Ministry of Health, 1944) that decisions of policy concerning the service should be made by accountable, elected representatives. A Central Health Services Council was subsequently established, allowing for the representation of professional expertise (Klein, 1989). Many hospital consultants opposed the greater state control that nationalisation of the service would bring about, by making them salaried employees. However conciliatory gestures by Bevan included the continued right of specialists to treat private patients in NHS hospitals (Klein, 1989). Similarly settlement with general practitioners was finally reached in favour of retention of their self-employed status, with further remuneration by capitation fees (Jones, 1994). Doctors effectively resisted attempts to draw them completely into a new bureaucratic hierarchy. Nevertheless nationalisation of health services posed a significant threat to medical autonomy as, prior to the NHS, no hospital had a boss and no doctor had a manager (Strong and Robinson, 1990). A more detailed account of the process of creating the NHS can be found in Chapter 3.

Despite great commitment by many to the philosophy of a service that was to be universal and free at the point of delivery, the settlement that ultimately produced the NHS conceded to medical power in ways that were to haunt the service for many years to come. As Smith (1993) suggests, the arrangements allowed the establishment of a core policy community consisting of the Ministry of Health, the Royal Colleges and the BMA which was responsible for overall health policy. Other professional groups were involved in a more exensive policy network and allowed access to policy making for specific issues only. The profession's close involvement with national health policy making reflected the ways doctors were able to achieve dominance over resources, expertise and knowledge. In particular doctors were able to influence policy through their ability to determine priorities, as well as successfully defining areas as professional issues, which they alone were qualified to manage (Klein, 1989). This is exemplified by the fervent and impassioned debate at the time, in the *British Medical Journal*, following the National Health Service Act, 1946 and leading to the settlement that eventually became the service in 1948. However, as Klein (1989) argues, the power of the profession, rather than being in its ability to impose its will, lay in its ability to block change, through the threat of withdrawal of support, a strategy redeployed by doctors in subsequent and more recent dealings with radical policy makers. Nevertheless, inevitably enshrined in the compromises that had become the NHS, major divisions from the past were perpetuated. These included the power of hospital consultants, the fragmentation of general practice and community and long-term care. Nursing, midwifery and other allied semi-professions remained subordinate and comparably impotent against medical dominance. Friction between local and central control, and between professional and bureaucratic power, subsequently gave rise to conflicts.

Throughout the early decades of the NHS, medical dominance was maintained. Klein (1989) has argued that medical authority became synonymous with the service and was institutionalised in ways that enabled the profession to control management, through presenting definitions of issues that reinforced their own authority. However, during this time, the state was able to exploit its position as a near monopoly employer of medical labour and thus was able to exert a downward pressure on salaries, compared with, for example, those of doctors in private sector health care in the United States. Nevertheless the medical profession permeated the decision making processes at all levels of the service and effectively achieved a right of veto over policy (ibid.).

The profession continued to use its power over other health professionals to influence health policy throughout the 1950s and 1960s. Medical authority became synonymous with the service, for example through medical advisory committees whereby doctors were able to determine priorities and successfully define areas as professional issues which only they were qualified to manage (ibid.).

Attempts to grapple with the inherited problems of the service, local versus central control, professional power versus bureaucratic power and in particular to constrain the power of the medical profession were made during the 1970s, 1980s and 1990s by successive governments in increasingly radical reorganisations of the service. As far back as 1954, the Bradbeer Report had considered the internal management of hospitals, raising concerns regarding the separate loyalties and hierarchies of occupational groups. In particular the

Report highlighted conflict between lay and medical administration, and recommended that, in order to strengthen management processes, all senior managers should be accountable to the employing authority through the chief administrative officer. In many ways Bradbeer represented an early precursor to the Griffiths Report.

The first reorganisation of the service came in 1974 after a series of consultative papers. Three managerial tiers were established at regional, area and district level. The new arrangements also introduced into the service a new corporate structure and management ethos, based on business lines (Strong and Robinson, 1990). Consensus management by teams of professionals, administrators and treasurers, in theory a group of equals with each team member representing the interests of a different occupational group, was introduced (Cox, 1991). It was unrealistically intended that decisions by the teams would be unanimous (Carrier and Kendall, 1986). Consensus management reinforced incrementalism in decision making (see Chapter 2), with each member of the team having a veto (Harrison and Pollitt, 1994). It was to prove to be both cumbersome and time-consuming, and ultimately failed. The balance of power between the different occupational groups who had never, in fact, been equals had been significantly misrepresented (Strong and Robinson, 1990).

A further reorganisation in 1982 abolished the area health authorities. The aim was to create more efficient management at all levels. The reorganisation acknowledged the need for an effective medical contribution to the management process, but although health authorities were obliged to consult professionals, there was no legal requirement to set up professional advisory committees.

Attempts to control the power of the medical profession by government were clearly not a new phenomenon: the tight grip on services, budgetary control and spending held by the medical profession had been the target of successive governments since the Bevan era. In the 1980s, in a political climate of strong conservatism, demands for greater accountability and financial control within the service emerged. The first Thatcher government placed great significance on efficiency, value for money and a need to reduce bureaucracy in the public sector, with its attendant delays, waste and costs (Jobling, 1989). Significantly more radical policy solutions were soon to unfold.

The Griffiths Reorganisation, 1984

Following the Conservatives' general election victory in 1983, Britain entered an era of ardent conservatism and increasing radicalism. The government commissioned Roy Griffiths, the managing director of Sainsbury's supermarket chain, to produce a report on the management of the NHS. The Griffiths Report was subsequently published on 25 October 1983. It proved to be the greatest challenge to 35 years of medical dominance since the inception of the service.

The philosophy of the Report was based on the belief that the commercial sector had a range of skills that could be of use in the NHS to facilitate enhanced management practice (Small, 1989). The changes recommended were designed to provide improved and dynamic leadership, at both macro and micro-management levels, motivate staff to maximise their potential and provide a more cost-effective service and greater value for money. Petchey (1986) has argued that considering the predominantly commercial and private sector background of the inquiry team, it was no surprise that their findings when made public, coincided precisely with governmental concern over the failure of cost containment measures. In particular one of the main findings of the Report was that there was a substantial failure of management, due to weak, ineffective consensus management (Harrison *et al.*, 1990).

The recommendations of the Report, which were implemented in 1984, advocated a new structure of management based on a commercial management model and drawn from within the 1982 reorganisation. This would include a general manager who would hold overall responsibility for the delivery of health services at unit, district and regional level. Regional general managers were to be responsible to an NHS Management Board and ultimately a Health Supervisory Board, to be chaired by the Secretary of State. Thus there was to be a direct line of accountability from unit level to the Secretary of State. The Griffiths recommendations therefore comprised an attempt to limit medical power through an increased bureaucratisation of the services with one individual, for the first time potentially not a medical officer, controlling each level. The voice of professionals was still to be heard, but rather in an advisory capacity which general managers might or might not heed. Administrators, whose role had been primarily as support for powerful professional groups, became managers, with responsibility for leadership and budgetary control, adopting an entrepreneurial style with the objective of improving efficiency and effectiveness. This theoretically left professionals, whom Griffiths regarded as 'resources to be managed', free to carry out their duties (Petchey, 1986).

Initially the health professions were largely distrustful of the proposals contained within the Griffiths Report and generally remained so. In particular they were concerned that their professional interests would be marginalised and that they would increasingly be dominated by health managers (Baggott, 1994). The immediate impact of the Griffiths reforms fell principally on the nursing profession. Griffiths himself had emphasised the importance of managers involving professionals in decision making (Klein, 1989), but with the demise of consensus management nurse managers in particular were to lose much of their power. Although the initial nursing response to the Report had been hostile, ultimately nurses co-operated in the hope of 'containing the fall out' (Petchey, 1986). Many of them, nevertheless, 'rose from the ashes' to be placed in charge of quality assurance (Klein, 1989). Petchey suggests that their intention had been to limit the consequences by ensuring that as many nurses as possible became general managers. Despite this the majority of new managers were drawn from the ranks of old-style administrators (Petchey, 1986).

The initial medical response to the Report was relatively restrained. The BMA suggested that, if the result would be to improve management, concentrate resources and reduce interference from the DHSS, doctors should welcome it (Petchey, 1986). The BMA subsequently negotiated the possibility of part-time managerial appointments for consultants, with resumption of clinical duties on completion of managerial contracts (ibid.). In addition some senior clinicians came to be involved in management as 'clinical directors' holding budgetary control and managerial responsibility for their unit or 'directorate', as well as for the management of medical colleagues.

The introduction of the general management function invariably led to a clash of occupational cultures (Small, 1989). Professional groups continued to see themselves as accountable principally to their own professional bodies, such as the BMA or the UKCC, (United Kingdom Central Council of Nursing, Midwifery and Health Visiting) and to patients, rather than line managers in an increasingly bureaucratic organisational culture. Following Griffiths, professional groups have been drawn into a bureaucratic hierarchy and have become answerable to senior management within that hierarchy. However the creation of a new cadre of professionals, the managers, may also be seen to increase the extent to which the service is made up of disparate occupational groups outside the bureaucratic framework, each with their own hierarchial structure and channels of accountability.

New management arrangements in the NHS have also led to the devolution of some power and decision making to unit level, but tensions between local decision making and tight central control have persisted into the 1990s as local people have demonstrated their objections to unpopular policies and decisions. Examples include the overwhelming opposition by Londoners to hospital closures following the publication of the Thomlinson Report (1992).

As a result of the Griffiths reforms the dominant paradigm of biomedicine has therefore been significantly challenged by that of financial accountability and management science. This has also attacked old-style administrative inefficiency and waste as well as the restrictive practices of the medical profession (Cox, 1992). Doctors for the first time have become answerable to a single postholder in the occupational hierarchy, with budgetary control and performance indicators designed to limit their power.

The Rise of the Professional Manager

Following Griffiths, a new professional occupational group has been seen to emerge in the NHS: the 'professional' manager. The phenomenon has been part of the wider Conservative government's strategy within the public sector of 'New Managerialism' (Davidson, 1987). The rationale has been to tighten and strengthen the managerial process, through increased rationalism in management, challenges to professional dominance and the provision of a more cost effective service. Harrison (1988) has argued that, up to the early 1980s, NHS management held a relatively weak and supportive position in relation to doctors. It was largely administrative, being concerned with servicing the needs of the professional, rather than with taking overall responsibility for the delivery of the service (Cox, 1991). Harrison (1988) further argues that, prior to Griffith, health management, rather than leading, was reactive, incremental and introverted.

It had developed largely within an ethos of public accountability in a context in which the medical profession held a pivotal position, principally aimed at maintaining the status quo rather than seeking change (Ranade, 1994). Harrison and Pollitt sum up the pre-1982 NHS manager as the 'diplomat' (1994); rather than shaping the service and controlling it, the manager 'helped to mediate conflicts' (1994: 36). Such a weak management style facilitated the maintenance of power by dominant professional groups.

Since Griffiths the new style NHS management has adopted scientific approaches to the management process. Nevertheless managers themselves can be seen to embody certain key characteristics or 'traits' of a profession. These include codes of conduct, a professional body such as the Institute of Health Service Management (IHSM), a period of education, for example the NHS Management Training Scheme, an NHS 'in house' fast track training scheme for managers, as well as higher education in professional subjects such as Masters in Business Administration (MBA). Nevertheless, despite increasingly developing as a professional group themselves, they remain one over which the government has been able to maintain tight control in ways it never achieved over other health professionals. Managers, for example, may be appointed on fixed term contracts with performance-related pay. They are subject to direction from an NHS hierarchy headed by the Secretary of State, who maintains a veto over appointments. Management activity is therefore tightly controlled from the centre by government, in order to ensure implementation of NHS policy. Thus, while post-Griffiths NHS managers may be seen to be the new professional group with considerable power over other groups, nevertheless their control by, and accountability to, government have set them apart from other professional groups.

Professional Power in the 1990s

Despite the rise of general management in the National Health Service, evidence of its impact on professionals suggests that at least up to the late 1980s, there had been little fundamental shift in the balance of power (Harrison *et al.*, 1992). Many clinicians came to be involved in management processes as clinical directorates enabled them to have a foothold in management while continuing to provide clinical services. Thus the rationale to involve doctors in management in order to seek their co-operation meant that many were able to hold on to much of their power. However more recent changes have given managers additional tools to help challenge medical hegemony.

Further reforms of the service, stemming from the NHS and Community Care Act 1990, addressed what Hunter has termed the 'unfinished business' at the 'medicine management interface' (1994: 5). Opportunities to monitor performance and clinical outcomes and to increase clinicians' financial accountability were seen as 'the last un-managed frontier of the NHS' (ibid.: 6). One of the major changes of the reforms was to divide the service into purchaser and provider functions. Hospital consultants, in particular, were situated in the provider camp. This in theory afforded an inducement for them to offer increasingly efficient, consumer-oriented services. This purchaser–provider split was imposed following closed, cabinet-level deliberations despite massive protest from doctors and opposition parties, as evidenced in poster campaigns and correspondence in medical journals at the time. Doctors were united in their anger at the government's failure to seek their advice and wisdom. Ministers had, in effect, terminated the practice of policy formation by consultation with the profession, thus ending a political relationship which has been described by Rhodes as typifying a 'professional network' (Rhodes, 1988).

The reforms posed a significant threat to the power and dominance of the medical profession. No longer would monolithic, producer-oriented policies be tolerated within the service. The powerful hospital consultants, whose presence on decision-making committees had previously significantly shaped resource allocation, had to bid for the contracts that determined service provision. Fundholding GPs and health commissioners would negotiate contracts with providers, on behalf of patients, based on local needs. In practice, fundholding GPs have tended to continue to use the services of providers with which they had previous links, thus not initially creating any dramatic changes in the distribution of resources (Klein, 1995).

The creation of purchasers and providers placed GPs in a more powerful position, both as fundholders and as non-fundholders, through their relationships with their health commissioner. GPs, in effect, now have a role in monitoring the performance of their hospital consultant colleagues as contracts for services become increasingly sophisticated, with purchasers seeking efficiency savings, improvements in waiting list conditions and Patient's Charter standards. Similarly the emphasis on developing primary care and preventive strategies, set out in the White Paper, *The Health of the Nation* (1992), has enhanced the role of public health doctors. Therefore, although the medical profession has never, in reality, constituted a homogeneous group, the reforms emphasised some significant divisions.

Further constraints on the medical profession brought about by the 1990 Act included the extension of the Resource Management Initiative. This had been piloted in 1987, with the intention of controlling spending by making doctors accountable for their budgets, assessing quality and providing information for management on the costs of clinical activity (Packwood *et al.*, 1991). Similarly medical audit, designed to provide self and peer appraisal and raise professional standards, which had previously been a voluntary exercise, became compulsory for hospital doctors and general practitioners, further extending their accountability. Klein has suggested, however, that medical audit has not been a total victory for management. The profession was able successfully to deflect the possibility of it becoming a powerful 'tool of management', as it sought to gain the initiative through internal regulation by medical peers (Klein, 1995: 244). This produced what Harrison and Pollitt have termed a 'medical model of medical audit' (1994: 101).

Other challenges since the 1990 Act through increased managerial and government control have begun to further 'invade the secret garden of professional discretion' (Klein, 1989: 211). The first of these include changes to GP contracts. These changes, also introduced in 1990, were imposed without the agreement of GPs. New contracts included payments for achieving targets for key services such as cervical screening and immunisation. Further payments were dependent on the provision of health promotion services such as Well Woman Clinics and health checks for elderly people. These alterations to GP renumeration meant that the amount of income generated from capitation fees rose from an average of just over 40 per cent to 60 per cent (Harrison and Pollitt, 1994). The rationale was to increase consumer power by creating greater incentives for GPs to compete for and retain patients and thus be more sensitive to their preferences.

Changes have also been imposed on hospital consultants' conditions of service. In particular these include an increased involvement of senior managers in deciding doctors' merit awards, consultant

appointments and job descriptions as a result of a widespread attempt
to replace professional or provider-driven services with tighter management control and services more responsive to consumer preferences (Hunter, 1991). Employment contracts, which had previously
been held at regional level, were devolved to local and trust levels
(Klein, 1995). Similarly changes to the criteria for consultant merit
awards have meant that consultants now have to demonstrate not
only clinical skills, but also their commitment to management (ibid.).
Waiting list initiatives have further confronted the disparity in work
practices between individual consultants (Yates, 1987; Klein, 1989).

The increased use of performance indicators (PIs) has also provided a challenge to the nature of the relationships between managers
and professional groups. For example, the publication of hospital
'league tables' in 1994 provided a star rating system for hospitals'
performance in key areas. These included the percentage of patients
admitted to hospital within three months and 12 months of being
placed on a waiting list. PIs have not, however, as yet, had a
significant impact upon the power base of the medical profession.
Harrison and Pollitt (1994) have argued that PIs have tended to be
used in a reactive rather than strategic manner, sustaining existing
policies rather than imposing new, more radical ones. They further
argue that some professionals have even been able to use them to
demand additional resources for their services. Government ministers
have made it clear that comparisons of how successfully doctors treat
patients will follow through, for example, the planned introduction of
performance-related pay for doctors (Hall, 1994). Furthermore criticism of increased bureaucracy and spiralling management costs in the
service may mean that managers themselves become victims of the
'friendly fire' of their own statistics. For example, PIs may well be
used in the future, to measure the performance of managers. Already
critics of the government are condemning what they see as the
increase in bureaucracy that the reforms have heralded. The *Guardian*
newspaper claimed in October 1995 a 400 per cent increase in health
managers over the previous five years, a 15 per cent increase in the
previous year, with some trusts spending over 10% of their budgets
on management.

In the same year a battle was fought, but not won, by nurses'
unions in a dispute with the government following an attempt to end
the Whitley Council national pay review body for health professionals. The majority of trusts eventually paid nurses the 3 per cent

recommended by the Pay Review Board. A further study in 1996 by the Incomes Data Services, however, highlighted the fact that, while nurses' pay rose an average of 3.2 per cent in the previous year, chief executives' pay had risen an average of 7.6 per cent. The trend towards the use of PIs in the service seems set to increase and the principle of local pay awards appears likely to become policy – both despite opposition from professionals' groups.

Finally threats to professional autonomy have arisen as measures to fragment and 'proletarianise' clinical tasks have been addressed by Regional Task Forces who, following *The New Deal* (DoH, 1991), have sought to redefine certain clinical tasks in an effort to reduce junior doctor hours. Such tasks, traditionally performed by doctors, may be taken on by other health professionals. Similarly, with regard to the nursing profession, managerial commentators such as Eric Caines have suggested that increased effectiveness and efficiency will be gained by 'cleaving off' some basic nursing tasks to other workers, namely those with cheaper skills (Davis, 1995). This might include, for example, the new 'support worker' role.

The Griffiths reorganisation may be seen as a watershed in the government's dealings with powerful professional groups in the NHS. Further challenges followed with the implementation of the NHS and Community Care Act 1990. Subsequent attempts by the government to tackle 'poorly performing doctors' and other groups through further challenges seem set to ensure further confrontation. In the mid-1990s, a time of increasing unpopularity of the Conservative government, ministers and health service managers have become the targets of unfavourable publicity. Condemnation has come from the government's critics and the media who have highlighted the high salaries and perks of senior managers, representing money that might, it is argued, be better be spent on patient care. In response to these criticisms, Stephen Dorrell, the Conservative Health Minister, announced at the party conference in 1995 new curbs on NHS management costs. This indicates that managers may themselves now become victims of challenges to professional power, in similar ways to those that other health professions have experienced. In the new style NHS, conflict between managers and professionals appears set to continue as professional groups seek to hold on to their power. However, as Klein (1995) has argued, the common interest which health professionals and managers have in the continuance of the institution and the services it provides may ultimately lead to co-operation.

Conclusions

This chapter has examined a range of traditional and critical approaches to the professions. It has explored the rise of medical power and the profession's ability to privilege itself over other groups of health workers and to influence health policy. It has also examined recent more radical approaches to health policy. In particular, following the Griffiths Report, new management arrangements posed a direct challenge to medical power. On the one hand, general management has led to an increased bureaucratisation of the service, as professional groups are drawn into an increasingly hierarchical occupational structure. On the other hand, however, there has emerged a new, powerful occupational group, the professional managers, with many of the 'traits' of a profession. Despite this, through fixed term contracts and performance-related pay, managers have less autonomy over their work than other professional groups. Tight central control is therefore maintained by government. More recent policy reforms following the NHS and Community Care Act 1990 have further challenged the power of the professionals. Although key groups such as the medical profession have maintained a strong power base in the service, recent policy statements have indicated that more radical measurement of professionals' performance, with increased managerial scrutiny of clinical practice, will follow. Similarly in the future managers themselves may be the target of scrutiny by government and subject to challenges to their power. This may lead to a climate of co-operation and interdependence as managers and professional groups recognise the need for each other in order to survive in the new organisational culture of the NHS.

Bibliography

Alleway, L. (1985) 'No Rush of New Blood Into the NHS', *Health and Social Services Journal*, vol. xcv, no. 4964, 12 Sept, p. 1121.
Baggott, R. (1994) *Health and Health Care in Britain*, Basingstoke: Macmillan.
Bleir, R. (1988) *Feminist Approaches to Science*, New York: Pergamon Press.
Carrier, J. and Kendall, I. (1986) 'NHS Management and the Griffiths Report', in M. Brenton and C. Ungerson (eds), *The Year Book of Social Policy in Britain*, London: Routledge & Kegan Paul.

Cox, D. (1991) 'Health Service Management – A Sociological View: Griffiths and the non-negotiated order of the hospital', in J. Gabe, M. Clanan and M. Bury (eds), *The Sociology of the Health Service*, London: Routledge.

Cox, D. (1992) 'Crisis and Opportunity in health Service Management', in R. Loveridge and K. Starkey (eds), *Continuity and Crisis in the NHS*, Buckingham: Open University Press.

Crompton, R. (1987) 'Gender, Status and Professionalism', *Sociology*, vol. 21, pp. 413–28.

Davidson, N. (1987) *A Question of Care: The Changing Face of the National Health Service*, London: Michael Joseph.

Davis, C. (1995) *Gender and the Professional Predicament in Nursing*, Buckingham: Open University Press.

DHSS (1983) *NHS Management Enquiry* (The Griffiths Report), London: DHSS.

Dingwall, R. (1994) 'Litigation and the Threat to Medicine', in J. Gabe, D. Keller and G. Williams (eds), *Challenging Medicine*, London: Routledge.

DoH (1991) *The New Deal*, London: HMSO.

DoH (1992) *Report of the Inquiry into London's health service, medical education and research* (The Thomlinson Report), London: HMSO.

DoH (1992) *The Health of the Nation*, London: HMSO.

Doyal, L. (1979) *The Political Economy of Health*, London: Pluto.

Ehrenreich B. and English, D. (1979) *For Her Own Good: 150 Years of the Experts' Advice to Women*, London: Pluto.

Elston, M. A. (1991) 'The politics of professional power: medicine in changing health service', in J. Gabe, M. Clanan and M. Bury (eds), *The Sociology of the Health Service*, London: Routledge.

Etzioni, A. (1969) *The Semi Professions and their Organisation*, New York: Free Press.

Fitzgerald, L. (1991) 'Made to Measure', *Health Service Journal*, 31 October, pp. 24–5.

Foster, P. (1989) 'Improving the Doctor/Patient Relationship: A Feminist Perspective', *Journal of Social Policy*, vol. 18, no. 3, pp. 337–61.

Fox, N. (1992) *The Social Meaning of Surgery*, Buckingham: Open University.

Freidson, E. (1970) *The Profession of Medicine*, New York: Harper & Row.

Giddens, A. (1989) *Sociology*, Cambridge: Polity Press.

Glazer, P. M. and Slater, M. (1987) *Unequal Colleagues: the entrance of women into the professions, 1890–1940*, New Brunswick and London: Rutgers University Press.

Greenwood, E. (1957) 'Attributes of a Profession', *Social Work*, vol. 2, no. 3, pp. 44–55.

Hall, D. (1994) *The Independent*, 20 July.

Harrison S. (1988) *Managing the National Health Service: Shifting the Frontier?* London: Chapman & Hall.

Harrison, S. and Pollitt, C. (1994) *Controlling the Professionals*, Buckingham: Open University.

Harrison, S., Hunter, D. and Pollitt C. (1990) *The Dynamics of British Health Policy*, London: Unwin Hyman.

Harrison, S., Hunter, D. J., Marnoch, G. and Pollitt, C. (1992) *Just Managing: Power and Culture in the National Health Service*, London: Macmillan.

Hugman, R. (1991) *Power in the Caring Professions*, London: Macmillan.

Hunter, D. J. (1991) 'Managing Medicine: A Response to the "Crisis"', *Social Science and Medicine*, vol. 32, no. 4, pp. 441–9.

Hunter, D. J. (1994) 'From Tribalism to Corporatism: the managerial challenge to medical dominance', in J. Gabe, D. Keller and G. Williams (eds), *Challenging Medicine*, London: Routledge.

Illich, I. (1976) *Limits to Medicine*, London: Calder & Boyars.

Jewson, N. (1976) 'The disappearance of the sick man from medical cosmology', *Sociology*, vol. 10, pp. 225–44.

Jobling, R. (1989) 'Health Care', in P. Brown and R. Sparks (eds), *Beyond Thatcherism, Social Politics and Society*, Milton Keynes: Open University Press.

Johnson, T. (1972) *Professionals and Power*, London: Macmillan.

Johnson, T. (1977) 'The Professions in the Class Structure', in R. Scase (ed.), *Industrial Society: Class Cleavage and Control*, London: Allen & Unwin, pp. 93–110.

Johnson, T. (1982) 'The State and the Professions: Peculiarities of the British', in A. Giddens and G. Mackenzie (eds), *Social Class and the Division of Labour*, Cambridge: Cambridge University Press, pp. 186–208.

Jones, H. (1994) *Health and Society in Twentieth Century Britain*, London: Longman.

Klein, R. (1989) *The Politics of the NHS*, London: Longman.

Klein, R. (1995) *The New Politics of the NHS*, London: Longman.

Kohler Reissman, C. (1989) 'Women and Medicalisation: A New Perspective', in P. Brown (ed.), *Perspectives in Medical Sociology*, Prospect Heights, CA: Wadsworth.

Kreckel, R. (1980) 'Unequal Opportunities Structure and Labour Market Segmentation', *Sociology*, vol. 4, pp. 525–50.

Kuznets, S. and Friedman, M. (1945) *Income from Independent Practice*, Washington: National Bureau of Economic Research.

Leap, N. and Hunter, B. (1993) *The Midwives' Tale: an oral history from handywoman to professional midwife*, London: Scarlet Press.

Martin, E. (1989) *The Woman in the Body*, Milton Keynes: Open University Press.

McKinlay, J. and Arches, J. (1985) 'Towards the Proletarianisation of Physicians', *International Journal of Health Services*, vol. 15, pp. 161–95.

Miles, A. (1988) *Women and Mental Illness*, London: Harvester Wheatsheaf.

Millerson, G. L. (1964) *The Qualifying Association*, London: RKP.

Ministry of Health (1944) *A National Health Service*, London: HMSO.

Moore, L. J. and Clarke, A. E. (1995) 'Clitoral Conventions and Transgressions: Graphic Representations in Anatomy Texts, c1900–1991', *Feminist Studies*, vol. 21, no. 2.

Navarro, V. (1976) *Medicine Under Capitalism*, New York: Prodist.

Oakley, A. (1984) *The Captured Womb, A History of the Medical Care of Pregnant Women*, Oxford: Basil Blackwell.

Oakley, A. (1993) *Essays on Women, Medicine and Health*, Edinburgh: Edinburgh University Press.

Oppenheimer, M. (1973) The Proletarianisation of the Professional, *Sociological Review Monograph*, vol. 20, pp. 213–37.

Packwood, T., Keen, J. and Buxton, M. (1991) *Hospitals in Transition. The Resource Management Experiment*, Buckingham: Open University Press.

Parkin, F. (1979) *Marxism and Class Theory: A Bourgeois Critique*, London: Tavistock.

Parry, N. and Parry, J. (1976) *The Rise of the Medical Profession*, London: Croom Helm.

Parsons, T. (1939) 'The Professions and the Social Structure', *Social Forces*, vol. 17, pp. 457–67.

Parsons, T. (1951) *The Social System*, London: Routledge & Kegan Paul.

Parsons, T. (1954) 'The Professions and Social Structure', in *Essays in Sociological Theory*, New York: Free Press.

Perkin, H. (1989) *The Rise of Professional Society: England Since 1880*, London: Routledge.

Petchey, R. (1986) 'The Griffiths reorganisation of the National Health Service', *Critical Social Policy*, vol. 17, no. 2, pp. 87–101.

Ranade, W. (1994) *A Future for the NHS?: Health Care in the 1990s*, London: Longman.

Rhodes, R. A. W. (1988) *Beyond Westminster and Whitehall*, London: Unwin Hyman.

Saks, M. (1994) 'The Alternatives to Medicine', in J. Gabe, D. Keller and G. Williams (eds), *Challenging Medicine*, London: Routledge.

Salmon, B. (1966) *Report of the Committee on Senior Nursing Structure*, London: HMSO.

Savage, W. (1986) *A Savage Inquiry: Who Controls Childbirth?*, London: Virago.

Scully, D. and Bart, P. (1978) 'A funny thing happened on the way to the orifice: the depiction of women in gynaecology textbooks', in J. Ehreinreich (ed.), *The Cultural Crisis of Modern Medicine*, New York: Monthly Review Press.

Small, N. (1989) *Politics and Planning in the National Health Service*, Milton Keynes: Open University Press.

Smith, M. J. (1993) *Pressure, Power, and Policy*, London: Harvester Wheatsheaf.

Stacey, M. (1988) *The Sociology of Health & Healing*, London: Routledge.

Strong, P. and Robinson, J. (1990) *The NHS Under New Management*, Milton Keynes: Open University.

Turner, B. (1987) *Medical Power and Social Knowledge*, London: Sage.

Ussher, J. (1991) *Women and Madness: Misogyny or Mental Illness*, Hemel Hempstead: Harvester Wheatsheaf.

Weber, M. (1949) *The Methodology of the Social Sciences*, New York: Free Press.

Witz, A. (1992) *Professions and Patriarchy*, London: Routledge.

Yates, J. (1987) *Why Are We Waiting?*, Oxford: Oxford University Press.

Zola, I. K. (1972) 'Medicine as an Institution of Social Control: The Medicalising of Society', *The Sociological Review*, vol. 20, no. 4, pp. 487–504.

6

Markets and Choice

Graham Moon

As Chapter 1 showed, central to the New Right health policy agenda during the first two Thatcher governments was a belief that private sector disciplines needed to be imposed on the NHS. Health was not alone in being a target for this neo-liberal prescription: other 'public' sector services received similar attention. Nor did health receive particularly intensive attention, perhaps as a consequence of the considerable public attachment to the service. The net consequence was, however, twofold. First, by the end of the 1980s, health policy had been affected by creeping privatisation (Haywood and Ranade, 1989): contracting had been introduced for some ancillary services and charges for some activities. Second, the basis for these developments had been located in a general concern for a version of efficiency in which the commonplace term 'value-for-money' had assumed centre stage. This second tendency had led, *inter alia*, to the introduction of general management, the abolition of area health authorities and the notion of the 'cost-improvement programme'. The two tendencies were, of course, clearly interlinked: privatisation was seen as umbilically entwined with efficiency, indeed, to all intents and purposes, private was efficient.

This brief synopsis does little justice to almost a decade of political history. Nor does it capture the considerable achievement of the Thatcherite project as it first introduced and then commenced the implementation of a neo-liberal view of social policy. It does, however, demonstrate that a degree of change already had been visited upon the NHS prior to the reforms of 1989/90; the notion of privatisation had been introduced and the constraints of money supply had been made clear. Notwithstanding the role of media and medical pressure in the immediate genesis of the reforms, the central question of the late 1980s was therefore the nature of the systemic change which had become inevitable. The disciplines of the market may have been imposed upon the actors and components of the system, but the system itself remained largely the same as that inherited by the Conservatives in 1979. This chapter takes as its subject matter the systemic reform of British health care policy which took place in the late 1980s and 1990s following the White Paper, *Working for Patients* (Secretary of State for Health, 1989). The chapter specifically considers the theoretical constructs which underpinned and informed the policies which were developed and commences with a general discussion of the pivotal idea of the 'market'. Attention then shifts to an analysis of the related construct of need. This conceptual discussion is cross-referenced, where appropriate, to the practicalities of the NHS reforms. The chapter then continues with an examination of the implications of the reforms for theories of policy implementation, before concluding with a brief consideration of the evolutionary or revolutionary nature of the reforms.

Markets

Thatcherism has been widely recognised as a complex phenomenon combining elements of neo-liberalism, neo-conservatism and populism (Gamble, 1988: Jessop *et al.*, 1988). Each of these tendencies is evident in the unfolding of health policy in the years following the 1989 White Papers, but it is perhaps neo-liberalism which provides, at least superficially, the clearest strategic backcloth. The neo-liberalism espoused by the Thatcher Conservatives was, of course, in evidence right from the start of their period of power and, in terms of political philosophy, was traceable back in time for at least two hundred years. Its key tenets were an emphasis on freedom, choice, the free market, minimal state intervention and the primacy of the individual (Joseph and Sumption, 1979). Of these characteristics, perhaps the most central is that of the free market.

Green (1987) has suggested that there are four strands or 'schools of thought' implicated in Thatcherite neo-liberalism: the Austrian (Hayek, 1960), the Chicago (Friedman, 1962), the Public Choice (Buchanan and Tullock, 1965; Niskanen, 1971) and the Anarcho-Capitalist (Nozick, 1974). In each the role of market is crucial. For Hayek, minimal state intervention and a free market was the situation most likely to create and encourage freedom through choice; government power should be limited so that the market may respond freely to consumer choice. The components of the market should stand or fall economically on their ability to satisfy the consumer. For Friedman, 'monetarism' indicated that the fiscal prudence of the providers of goods and services should actually shape the market; the state should play very much a residual role. The public choice theorists noted that the interests of those running state services were best served by having a large public sector; this they argued was inherently inefficient as it challenged the hegemony of the market. Where complete removal of the public sector was impossible, they argued for the introduction of pseudo-market discipline and constitutional limitations to the activities of public sector organisations. Public choice perspectives were of growing influence in Britain through the second Thatcher government. Finally, and of least importance in the British context, the anarcho-capitalists advocated unrestricted freedom, the abolition of the state and a grassroots democratic polity based on individual choice: an atomised market.

The market therefore became seen as a crucial requirement for the further development of Thatcherism; without a more marketised socioeconomic form of organisation, the privatisation initiatives which had begun to 'roll back the state' would founder on the rocks of a recalcitrant and entrenched public sector bureaucracy protecting and even enhancing its own interests and a consumer body characterised by a dependency culture. The market would provide the crucial context for fostering individual freedom because of its basis of choice and its encouragement to individuals to pursue their own self-interests. Yet the market would also mysteriously equilibrate these diverse interests through the notion of the 'invisible hand'. State interference in the market would thus not only undermine individual freedom, it would also damage societal organisation.

Pure free markets may have been, and continue to be, on the agenda for some radical conservative politicians; they certainly were and are on the agendas of right-wing think tanks such as the Institute for Economic Affairs and the Adam Smith Institute. However their implementation has been constrained by two forces. First, it has not proved easy to replace the Fabianist legacy of the post-Second World War consensus. A relatively substantial public sector had developed prior to the economic crisis of 1976 and sociopolitical expectations had become deeply ingrained. The second constraint to the implementation of the free market ideal was in a sense related to the first: the neo-conservative and populist aspects of Thatcherism militated against wholesale marketisation. From the neo-conservative perspective (Marsland, 1988), tradition, stability and authority were important; considerable respect was accorded to existing institutions and only a strong state was thought to be able to guarantee the effective and unfettered operation of the market. The consequence of this tendency was occasional protectionism and considerable centralisation. From the populist perspective (Mohan, 1995), Thatcherism sought, on the one hand, to demonise the public sector through the promotion of the idea of the 'nanny state' and to promote the virtues of self-reliance via private, family and community self-help. On the other hand, they faced the considerable support for public services and, in the specific case of the NHS, incontrovertible evidence (OECD, 1993) that it had proved to be the cheapest way of bringing mass effective health care to the electorate.

The nature of any market clearly reflects the institutional and political context in which it develops or is fostered (Hindess, 1987). For the Thatcherites, the constraints, both circumstantial and self-imposed, which they faced meant that a shift to a full-blown market economy was both politically and socially untenable. What was required was, in line with public choice theory, a means of exposing the public sector to market demands in a market-like context. Such a requirement entailed consideration of two matters: service funding and service organisation. The former would involve an assessment of the relative merits of tax, insurance and private funding for service provision. While Thatcherites might naturally gravitate towards the merits of private funding, the services on which their attention focused were traditionally and popularly provided on a tax-funded basis; change might have electoral consequences. Service organisation reform centred attention on the monolithic, anti-competitive, unitary nature of an unmarketised public sector. Here change was less problematic; what was possible was the fragmentation of the mono-lith, the introduction of competition *within* a still largely public sector and the encouragement of a more pluralist approach to service organisation. In short, though a free market was not possible, the Thatcherites could create a quasi-market (Bartlett, 1991; Bartlett and Le Grand, 1993; Bartlett and Harrison, 1993) in which managed competition could take place under the watchful eyes of the strong central state.

Marketising the NHS

Analyses of the 1989 NHS reforms are now legion. Readers seeking
detail should refer to Kendall and Moon (1990, 1994) for condensed
accounts or to the excellent interpretations of Ranade (1994), Klein
(1995) or Mohan (1995) for extended assessments. In this section
attention will simply be on the ways in which the Thatcherite project
sought to apply the concept of the quasi-market to the NHS; a full
exegesis of the reforms will not be presented. Nevertheless some detail
is necessary in order to appreciate the nature of the changes which
were introduced.

The genesis of the NHS reforms can be traced back several years
and certainly includes the introduction of general management and
the general facilitation of privatisation during the 1980s. More
immediately, however, the origin of the reforms lay in two distinct
areas. First, and almost perversely, the limitations of the earlier
initiatives had fostered a frustration on the part of those involved in
the implementation of change. The new managers were heavily
constrained by bureaucratic controls and perverse incentives which
limited their scope for introducing new measures aimed at greater
service efficiency (Strong and Robinson, 1990). As a consequence of
this frustration, a cadre of people existed who were within the NHS
but eager to continue the process of change. Second, 1987 saw the
NHS in one of its endemic funding crises. The acute (hospital) sector
attracted the most attention with wards being closed, operations
cancelled, payments delayed, reserves depleted and, most crucially,
prominent cases of young children suffering as a consequence of
cutbacks. The popular and professional opinion was that the NHS
was grossly underfunded. This did not chime, however, with political
opinion within the Conservative Party where the crisis was ascribed
to public sector profligacy, but, as 1987 was an election year, the
NHS enjoyed a short-term electoral bonus of additional funding
which was enough to diminish the crisis. No change was intimated
in the Conservatives' electoral manifesto; however, once they were
returned to power, the crisis showed every sign of returning. Again a
cash injection was made, but the opportunity was also seized to
review the NHS.

In a typically populist stroke, the formal start of the review, indeed
the first announcement of the review, was made by the Prime
Minister in a television interview. From the start, Margaret Thatcher

stamped her personality on the review. She chaired the meetings of the five-member review team and, though there is some evidence that the review lost momentum at one stage, was able to reimpose a degree of radicality on its conclusions when it finally came to report a year after its beginning. The assembled review team naturally included the Secretary of State for Health and Social Services, but was dominated by Treasury interests in reflection of the fiscal crisis which had precipitated its creation.

The agenda of the review was clearly concerned with value for money. Themes of equity which had inspired earlier reviews such as the Black Report (DHSS, 1980) and even the Royal Commission on the NHS (1979) were avoided. Consideration was to be limited to the fundamentals of neo-liberalism, to the possibilities of reforming the funding base and the organisation of the service. Not unsurprisingly, given the popular support for the existing tax-funded basis to the NHS, funding changes did not emerge, except in one minor sense. Alternatives were certainly considered. Vouchers, a favourite Fried-manite strategy, were one possibility, others were private or public health insurance schemes operating either individually or through some equivalent of the United States' 'health maintenance organisa-'tions' (HMOs), schemes which negotiate packages of care and to which individuals belong for a fee. Each would have had problems. Vouchers would have had technical difficulties – setting the value of the vouchers and arranging their distribution (Scheffler, 1989). Insurance schemes were known to drive up costs if they were to enable anything like the sort of universal cover expected by the British electorate (Fowler, 1991). HMOs were recognised as discriminatory and inegalitarian, again offending the principle of universalism (Petchey, 1987). As a result of the recognition of these problems, the NHS emerged from the review as a service which would continue to be funded from general taxation. The only innovation to creep in was the granting of tax relief on private health care insurance contributions to elderly people; Mohan (1995: 66) sees this as 'the triumph of ideology over rationality' and a not particularly covert attempt to favour core Conservative voters.

The reforms were therefore grounded in an unchanged funding base. Perceptions of a lack of funds were not considered and alternative ways of generating funds were not adopted. The reality of the reforms was a concern with reorganising the way the service worked. A particular form of quasi-market had to be evolved in which competition could be introduced to the NHS and, just possibly, costs driven down as consumers looked for cheaper but as effective options. The model for such a situation was the internal market (Enthoven, 1985). Enthoven's internal market posited the separation of the direct provision of health care (hospitals, clinics, surgeries and home nursing) from the initial purchasing of that care (planning levels of provision, resource allocation and distribution). Providers would work simply at caring for people with health problems. Purchasers would seek out providers who offered an acceptable compromise between cheapness, availability and adequate quality. Purchasers would be responsible for buying, from providers, care sufficient to satisfy the health care needs of their defined population. Providers would be free to sell their services to any purchaser; they would compete with other providers and endeavour to ensure that they addressed consumer needs at competitive prices. The whole system would be driven by a contracting process linking purchaser and provider in annually renegotiable agreements.

The internal market facilitated a number of transformative shifts in the NHS. First, the unitary service was split into two arms: purchasers and providers. The monolith was fragmented into two dissimilar operations. Initially both purchaser and provider functioned as arms of an overarching health authority. Rapidly, however, the health authority metamorphosed into the purchaser and the provider arms took up semi-independent 'trust' status. Second, market discipline was heightened. On the one hand, the purchaser–provider contract negotiations provided a means to set clear cost parameters and quality expectations after an initial period of stasis in which 'steady-state' arrangements were encouraged and the government sought to phase in the rigours of the market. On the other hand, individual providers had to compete with each other and respond to consumer demand as articulated by the purchasers. Third, purchasers could purchase where they wished, including the private sector. This had the effect of legitimising the position of the private sector. It also had the effect of radically damaging the traditional markets of some providers as more effective, often more local, solutions were sought. London hospitals and regional speciality providers in particular were strongly affected by the operation of the internal market as purchasers encouraged more accessible provision (Tomlinson, 1992). One of the criticisms of the internal market was that it might lead to purchasers buying cheap but distant care; paradoxically the actual outcome was an increasing duplication of resources at more local levels.

The position of the trust status providers within the internal market deserves some specific consideration. Although it was always stressed that trusts remained within the NHS, the initiative was clearly designed to stress the scope for entrepreneurialism which the Conservatives saw as integral to the reform of public service. Trusts were given self-governing status and were to be dependent on their success in attracting contracts from purchasers; they were to live and potentially die by the market. Unfortunately so too might their patients, as an all too clear correlation between fiscal health and patient care was possible. In cutting themselves free from local health authority control, trusts were to gain the right to set their own pay levels and conditions of service, decide their market and, if necessary and subject to conditions, raise capital for developments and dispose of unwanted assets. They were seen as simultaneously a manifestation of the attack on bureaucracy and a source of innovation. Furthermore, as quasi-businesses, they were expected to pursue an ethic of commercial confidentiality concerning their activities; public scrutiny of their meetings was to be limited. The trust therefore embodies the very essence of a neo-liberal quasi-market policy model: independent (in a sense), driven by the economics of the market and freed of the fetters of traditional control.

Before ending this focused analysis of the implementation of quasi-markets in the NHS, one further characteristic of that implementation needs to be noted. In pure free markets the consumer is sovereign. Such a situation does not happen in quasi-markets, nor did it happen in the specific case of the NHS. Consumers in the strict individualised sense gained little. Prior to the reforms they had had little choice about their treatment; after the reforms little changed regarding direct consumer choice. Purchasers in effect operated as proxy consumers. For a majority of conditions, the treatment choices for secondary care referrals by GPs were those identified by the local purchaser. For a minority of conditions, GPs themselves made those decisions, provided they were fundholders – practices which had been allocated a budget to purchase directly a restricted list of care procedures (Glennerster *et al.*, 1994). With primary care there had always of course been a choice, at least in urban areas, over which GP to register with. There had also always been an ostensible right to change GPs; it remained apparent rather than certain after the reforms. The nature of consumer choice in the NHS quasi-market was therefore somewhat restricted. What was incontrovertible, however, was the far greater role which a rhetoric of consumer sensitivity came to play in the years following the reforms.

In summary, the implementation of the quasi-market model in the NHS provided the Conservatives with a context in which neo-liberal policy options could be operationalised. This bald statement of course embodies many contradictions. The quasi-market was a compromise for some. The very idea of government implementing policy would offend some neo-liberals. Nevertheless the process brought freedom, market discipline, a fragmentation of a formerly unitary service and an injection of (a particular form of) consumerism. As will be argued later, the process was, of course, far from problem-free, nor was it without inherent flaws. For the moment, however, attention will turn to a perhaps paradoxical driving force of the reformed system: the concept of need.

Need

Need was central to the NHS when it was founded. Why should its continuing importance after 1989 be paradoxical? Quite simply, the logic of the market should imply that cost – or perhaps cost utility or efficiency – should replace need, a soft, outmoded Fabian concept of little relevance in a market-driven world. Yet need retained its importance. In part this was undoubtedly because of the historical resonance of the concept with a British public reared on the description of the NHS as a service predicated on the allocation of resources according to need. However it was also because the concept of need possessed certain chameleon-like characteristics which enabled it to be adapted and moulded to the requirements of the market. This section will explore notions of need, their implications for the NHS and their adaptation in the post-reform era.

The now well-established typology of Bradshaw (1972) provides an insight into the shifting and contestable nature of the concept of need that retains considerable usefulness. Bradshaw separated need into normative, felt, expressed and comparative aspects. Each resonates with the application of the concept of need within the NHS. Normative need raises the spectre of normative planning whereby need was addressed through crude, expert-defined planning norms such as the average list size of a GP or through complex variously adjusted formulae in the case of the pre-reform resource allocation process (DHSS, 1976). Felt need captures the underlying wants of the population of actual and potential NHS consumers. Expressed need sees those wants translated into a request for services: a demand. Comparative need introduces the politics of envy, 'this community needs a new hospital because that community has just had one', but it also contributes a reminder that simple comparative analysis demonstrates easily that the NHS did not bring about equality during its first 40 years (Townsend *et al.*, 1992). Of course, it may well be that none of these characterisations actually represents need in the strict sense. Norms, wants, demands, envy and inequality are all aspects of a matter which, as Bradshaw himself later noted, is inherently problematic in the case of the NHS (Bradshaw, 1994).

As a central plank of the welfare state, need was the subject of much intellectual controversy following the election of the Conservative government in 1979. Among the most influential general statements have been those of Doyal and Gough (1984, 1991). They have argued that a modern definition of need should be concerned with an individual's ability to participate in social life. The fundamental prerequisites of such participation are good physical health and personal autonomy, but these are not needs in themselves; need is the participatory opportunity. For the New Right, discussion concerning need centred upon the extent to which need could be reconciled with the tenets of neo-liberalism. Two general aspects to this reconciliation can be distinguished: the atomisation of needs and its equation with economic matters.

The first of these representations draws in the neo-liberal emphasis on the individual as opposed to the collective. Notions of universal services, the basic policy legacy of the welfare state, are rejected in favour of an individualised approach with needs satisfied via the market. Green (1986) argued, for example, that health care need was innately personal, being bound up with individual evaluations of pain, risk, potential disability and likelihood of death. He repudiated universalisation, a process by which individual needs could be submerged in some overall average approach in which no one member of the participating society would actually be satisfied. The New Right were also particularly suspicious of distinctions between relative and absolute need. While some adherents to the Friedmanite idea of a residual state might concede a need for some form of 'safety-netting' for those in absolute need, most would reject relative need, and with it some aspects of Bradshaw's comparative need, as simply a means of extending need to benefit the less deserving and facilitate the 'nanny state' (Harris, 1988).

It would be tempting to sum up the New Right's atomisation of need by suggesting that it meant that only individuals would be truly able to articulate their need. This would, however, neglect two further factors. First, as was noted in the previous section, the market systems which the Conservatives were able to introduce were not perfect: they were quasi-markets. Individual consumers did not come to exercise real sovereignty. Consumer needs were interpreted and mediated by professionals and by managers. Such interest groups were, in the New Right public choice analysis, likely to manipulate needs to the benefit of the organisation. This tendency had to be guarded against by objectifying the process of needs assessment to the greatest possible degree. Second, and notwithstanding the first problem, there also remained some doubt as to whether individuals, or their advocates, would be truly able to separate needs from demands or wants – or even, in a climate of consumer facilitation, preferences. This too resolved into a case for objectifying needs assessment.

The equation of need with economic matters is part of this process of objectification. Put simply, a key populist justification for much New Right policy during the 1980s was 'sound economic management'. The anticipated benefit of the introduction of quasi-markets was that they would bring a form of market efficiency to bear on the public sector. For the purchasers of services, it would be essential to turn away from demand management towards the meeting of 'real' need (almost from the beginning of the NHS it had been recognised that demands were infinite and incapable of satisfaction within a cash-limited service (Ministry of Health, 1956; Powell, 1966)). Such needs would have to be translated into contracts with providers and the effectiveness of providers would have to be assessed in terms of their relative success in meeting the needs. In a marketised system it was inevitable that cost would be attached to such matters. Isolating real need from demand was not a task which health economists had relished historically (Williams, 1978). They were, however, thoroughly conversant with such ideas as cost–benefit analysis, cost–utility analysis and cost–effectiveness analysis (Mooney, 1986). The development of quasi-markets represented an unparalleled disciplinary opportunity to apply these tools through identifying the cost of small improvements in people's health. This simultaneously injected a cost element into the internal market and provided an element of rationality to needs assessment.

Since the NHS reforms, the key to the continued importance of need has lain in the expectation that purchasers should buy health care for their resident population on the basis of that population's need for health care. The purchasers have thus had to address the task of unpacking the concept of need from the theoretical and philosophical positions set out in the preceding paragraphs; they have also had to operationalise need in the particular context of the neo-liberal vision. The providers have then had to accommodate the differing operationalisations of need of the various purchasers with which they deal. From the preceding paragraph it will have become clear that health economics is one element of this operationalisation. Health economics has been promoted as a rational means by which purchasers can decide between competing demands. By linking capacity to benefit with the cost of benefit, it purports to enable purchasers to address sticky questions of equity within the context of a quasi-market limited by central cash allocations. The relative impact of treating a few expensive cases or many cheaper cases, of investing in particular items of medical technology, of new therapies versus old – all can be addressed, at least in theory, by the techniques of health economics. In practice, of course, while it may help decision making, much subjectivity remains. While it may inject an element of rationality into a messy arena, the intertwining of demand and need therefore remains a problem.

To consider how the NHS quasi-market has addressed this issue, attention needs to turn to another professional group which grew in status in the years following the NHS reforms. Public health medicine had been an influential force in Victorian times, pointing to the links between poor housing, sanitation and levels of ill-health in the population. By the mid-1980s, however, its role had been substantially overshadowed by clinical curative medicine. The influential Acheson Report (DHSS, 1988) began a process of reinvention for the public health function but it was the advent of the internal market which really provided the speciality with a new *raison d'être*: public health medicine specialists were well placed to provide the new purchasers with seemingly objective advice about the need for health care. In the first place, public health medicine specialists had a training focused on epidemiological method and enquiry which fitted them superbly well to evaluate literature on competing treatment options and their outcomes; epidemiological work also underpinned much of the work which equated health need to mortality, morbidity and social pathology. Second, the public health medicine specialists were often the only people in a purchasing organisation with direct, certified clinical knowledge; they understood clinical literature and could converse with and convince other medical personnel. Furthermore, as a consequence of this position, they were able to offer purchasing decisions the stamp of the 'expert' decision. Finally public health directors were guaranteed places on boards of health authorities; their position in the hierarchy was assured. For the New Right, these matters brought medicine into the orbit of the internal market; they incorporated a group who might otherwise have been a strong opponent of the market with its potential to increase health inequalities. It also objectified the definition of need and gave it an aura of scientific rationality.

Public health thus came to assume an important role. This role enabled need to be objectively defined in terms of epidemiological information on morbidity and mortality; health care was to be bought to ensure reductions in such key indicators and the information was routinely provided in annual public health common data sets. Desired reductions were codified in the *Health of the Nation* White Paper (DoH, 1992), a document which set out a *health* policy as opposed to a *health care* policy and focused on a strongly biomedical analysis of a limited set of health problems. The strategies for achieving disease reductions were also strongly biomedical, reflecting the influence of the public health medicine specialists – as well as a public expectation that health care should be biomedical, curative and interventionist. Perhaps the key concept to emerge was that of evidence-based medicine (Sackett *et al.*, 1985): making clinical choices upon the basis of the cumulative indications of past epidemiological studies concerning improvements to health. Around this notion developed a whole industry of advisory services devoted to providing evidence in an acceptable form. These included the Cochrane Centres (named after an influential public health specialist who had called for economic evaluations of medical interventions (Cochrane 1972)), the Centre for NHS Reviews and Dissemination and a new journal, *Evidence-Based Medicine*.

In process terms, the revival of the public health role therefore centred on the public health departments taking on the task of needs assessment for purchasers. This work provided an underpinning to the process of contract setting through option selection and target assignment (EL(90)MB/86, 1990). For Stevens and Gabbay (1991) this approach was somewhat simplistic as it assumed, perhaps naively, that epidemiological definitions of need avoided the problem of the need–demand conflict; in reality the data on which they were based were seldom capable of making such precise separations. To improve the system, the Department of Health instituted a process of needs assessment based on supplementing epidemiological assessments with comparative and 'corporate' approaches. The first was similar to the definition of Bradshaw (1972), while the latter built upon notions of management target setting and ideas of achievable performance. Notwithstanding these official positions, the operationalisation of need has continued to be problematic.

One reason for this continuing difficulty has concerned the negative use value of need. Put crudely, while need can be used positively to identify and then satisfy people in need, it can also be used negatively with the definition of need being drawn so tightly that certain people are excluded from 'the needy' and health care becomes 'rationed'. In a cash-limited system like the NHS, the tendency for the negative definition to apply is considerable and it is not surprising that rationing is a well-established element of decision making in the NHS (Honigsbaum *et al.*, 1995). Traditionally, however, rationing happened when the budget ran out at the end of the financial year. Since the advent of the internal market, much greater financial control is possible. Some health authorities have contemplated experiments similar to that conducted in the state of Oregon in the USA where health commissioners and the public ranked diseases and associated treatments in terms of priority and refused to pay for the least popular. Most, however, have stuck with epidemiologically led needs definitions which have embodied clear evidence-based guidelines on the population groups most likely to benefit from particular treatments. This strategy has further cemented the central position of public health in needs assessment but at the same time it has meant that the public health specialists have become increasingly seen as the group most clearly responsible for the legitimation of rationing.

It would be dangerous to conclude this section by suggesting that need has been hijacked by the New Right and that the combined forces of the health economists and the public health specialists have been the agents of this operation. This would be a gross caricature and a cruel misrepresentation as need remains a very slippery concept and, certainly in the public health field, there are many who lament its use as a rationing instrument. Need did, however, manage to maintain its position as a key tenet of the NHS at a time when fiscal discipline was growing and the advent of purchasing demanded a more overtly rational conception of the concept. The interaction of these tendencies has led to considerable change in both the conception and the use of need.

Policy Implementation in a Quasi-Market

It will by now be evident that the marketisation of the NHS illustrates many of the general dilemmas concerning markets and welfare services which were suggested in the earlier part of this chapter. The public regard in which the unitary NHS, perhaps the key achievement of the post-Second World War welfare state, was held has already been noted. Notice should also be drawn to the respect accorded to health care workers, particularly doctors, as front-line providers of health care; their power and that of their representative organisations had to be taken into account in any shift in policy. To these problems of implementation must be added those difficulties which arise from the general weaknesses of the market approach and its application by the Conservatives.

The *Working for Patients* White Paper itself was a classic example of Thatcherite policy making (Mohan, 1995). It involved limited consultation within an inner circle of people committed to Thatcherite aims; submissions were not sought but where they were made they tended to come from interest groups within the health services and from right-wing think tanks. The latter were highly influential in establishing specific elements of the reforms, notably the inclusion of tax relief on private health insurance for elderly people and the notion of trust status. The public were not formally consulted, nor were health workers, though the latter submitted views. This tight, purposeful approach to policy making contrasts sharply with the more evolutionary, developmental and consultative approaches of previous years. It suggests that the key elements of the agenda were firmly established in the minds of those involved: neo-liberal arrangements were to be generated for the NHS in order to provide (cf.

Edelman, 1971) a symbolic gesture towards resolving the perceived inadequacies of the existing system.

Implementing *Working for Patients* required a huge commitment of time, energy and resources to shift the NHS from a unitary service to one organised on the basis of a purchaser–provider split. Such a change inevitably meant that past incrementalist approaches to change were discredited; as noted above in the discussion of need, rational decision making was, at least in theory, the chosen approach to policy implementation. The application of market principles carried with it a clear commitment to setting and meeting targets for the implementation of the system. Most of these targets were met; the major slippage occurred with community care, where parallel internal market arrangements were delayed for a year. Nevertheless the implementation targets were generally subject to staging as some elements of the NHS proved able to change more quickly than others. While few provider units took on trust status and few GPs went for fundholding initially, an increasing number subsequently made the changes. Furthermore rationalism had to accommodate the powerful interests of the clinicians whose continuing commitment remained essential.

In practice, the rationalist claims of the new system were therefore overlaid with a considerable residue of 'muddling through' as managers learnt the ropes of the new system and made judgements about how fast to proceed. The rationalist claims were also overshadowed by a realisation that, despite the arrival of managerialism in the NHS, the acquiescence of the health professions was still needed if the reforms were to 'work'. An element of interest group management had therefore to be retained despite the general New Right inclination to dismiss interest groups as self-interested lobbies. The growing role of the public health specialist and the ascendancy of epidemiological needs assessment undoubtedly represented part of this strategy of policy implementation through interest group management: incorporating an element of the medical profession and giving prominence to a medically derived concept of need contributed to the legitimation of the reforms in the eyes of the medical profession. This legitimation was also enhanced by the growing prominence of clinical directorates as a form of trust management and the surge in the numbers of GP fundholders. Though medical support for the reforms was never extensive, antipathy was thus never capable of developing into concerted and continued opposition.

In the process of implementing the internal market, further pressures for change naturally emerged as the impact of the market on the existing pattern of services became clearer. It has already been noted that, as time progressed, increasing numbers of providers in the primary, secondary and community fields effectively 'went to market' by becoming trusts or fundholders. It has also been noted that some providers found themselves jeopardised by the operation of the market: their services were no longer being bought in the volume needed to sustain existing operating levels. Thus rationalisation occurred in the London hospital scene as a consequence of purchasers taking their custom elsewhere. For purchasers, the market brought pressures to merge to create larger economies of scale and to unify to end the somewhat artificial divide between primary and secondary/community health care. District purchasers were also increasingly threatened by the growth of and subsequent plans for extending fundholding. The pressures of implementing a policy embedded in neo-liberalism were, however perhaps most keenly felt at regional level. Regions bore the brunt of a continuing conviction that the NHS was overburdened with bureaucrats and overprone to attempts to control the market; the regions were first merged and then reformulated as 'regional offices' of the NHS Executive. In this new and much slimmed-down guise they were to play a 'hands-off' monitoring role rather than interfere with the local operation of the market.

These diverse pressures and developments created a system in which no sense of emerging stability could be detected but a number of paradoxes and problems could. First, and paradoxically, despite attempts to represent the changing role of the regions to the contrary, the reforms actually encouraged centralisation. Such a finding is common to evaluations of many Thatcherite policy initiatives and suggests a realisation that markets require management if they are to be effective. Second, fundholding, arguably the most innovative of the reforms, provided a basis for the destruction of the universalist conception of the NHS; GP fundholders were able to buy better care for their patients. In market terms they simply provided a better service. Third, market discipline increased efficiency but, arguably, displaced the problem; in order to discharge patients quickly and keep NHS costs down, costs may have been shifted to social care budgets – or directly to the families or individuals involved. Fourth, the consumer has little genuine direct involvement in decision making, being still dependent on the knowledge and recommendations of the purchaser. Finally, it is of course, despite the NHS reforms, still by no means morally or ethically clear that health care is a commodity which can really be managed and delivered through a market. Markets naturally entail rationing, denial, exclusion and 'inability to afford'; it is not clear that quasi-markets incorporating residual commitments to welfarist goals can wholly avoid these problematic areas.

Conclusion

In introducing quasi-markets to the NHS arena, the Conservatives succeeded in extending their neo-liberal project. They provided the all-important context in which they could further develop a pre-existing commitment to roll back the state and restructure welfarism. The quasi-market was, however, not the free market that some might have wished for. It was a state regulated market in which professional interests had to be incorporated and popular concerns reconciled. Furthermore its operation and continued evolution were not possible without the development of a rational–scientific approach to needs assessment and a substantial element of central direction. The NHS reforms might therefore effectively be seen as a compromise in favour of practical and political expediency rather than a free market ambition.

This characterisation would imply that the NHS reforms were indeed reforms: they did not represent a revolutionary change. Such a conclusion would be correct. Moreover the reforms were also a point in a process of evolution. The Thatcher project had put in place many of the essential elements for the reforms some time before the publication of *Working for Patients*. The introduction of general management, increased prescription charging, primary care reform, the contracting out of ancillary work and the growth of the private sector had all taken place. A pluriform health care system in which private care co-existed with public and family care was already a fact of life. What was lacking was the market environment necessary for the further enhancement of these developments. The introduction of quasi-markets was thus a logical move. It was in accord with both the government's ideological preference and its record with other erst-while 'public' services.

Bibliography

Bartlett, W. (1991) 'Quasi-markets and contracts: a markets and hierarchies perspective on the NHS reforms', *Public Money and Management*, vol. 11, pp. 53–61.

Bartlett, W. and Harrison, L. (1993) 'Quasi-markets and National Health Service Reforms', in W. Bartlett and J. Le Grand (eds), *Quasi-Markets and Social Policy*, London: Macmillan.

Bartlett, W. and Le Grand, J. (1993) 'The theory of quasi-markets', in W. Bartlett and J. Le Grand (eds), *Quasi-Markets and Social Policy*, London: Macmillan.

Bradshaw, J. (1972) 'A taxonomy of social need', in G. McLachlan (ed.), *Problems and Progress in Medical Care*, Oxford: Oxford University Press.

Bradshaw, J. (1994) 'The conceptualisation and measurement of need: a social policy perspective', in J. Popay and G. Williams (eds), *Researching the People's Health*, London: Routledge.

Buchanan, J. and Tullock, G. (1965) *The Calculus of Consent*, Ann Arbor: University of Michigan Press.

Cochrane, A. (1972) *Effectiveness and Efficiency*, London: Nuffield Provincial Hospitals Trust.

DHSS (1976) *Sharing Resources for Health in England*, London: HMSO.

DHSS (1980) *Inequalities in Health: Report of a Research Working Group*, London: DHSS.

DHSS (1988) *Public Health in England: The Report of the Committee of Inquiry into the Future Development of the Public Health Function*, Cmnd 289, London: HMSO.

DoH (1992) *The Health of the Nation*, London: HMSO.

Doyal, L. and Gough, I. (1984) 'A theory of human needs', *Critical Social Policy*, vol. 4, pp. 6–38.

Doyal, L. and Gough, I. (1991) *A Theory of Human Need*, London: Macmillan.

Edelman, M. (1971) *The Politics of Symbolic Action*, Chicago: Markham.

EL(90)MB/86 (1990) *Developing Districts*, London: HMSO.

Enthoven, A. (1985) *Reflections on the Management of the NHS*, London: Nuffield Provincial Hospitals Trust.

Fowler, N. (1991) *Ministers Decide*, London: Chapman.

Friedman, M. (1962) *Capitalism and Freedom*, Chicago: University of Chicago Press.

Gamble, A. (1988) *The Free Economy and the Strong State: The Politics of Thatcherism*, London: Macmillan.

Glennerster, H., Matsaganis, M., Owens, P. and Hancock, S. (1994) *Implementing GP Fundholding*, Milton Keynes: Open University Press.

Green, D. (1986) *Challenge to the NHS: A Study of Competition in American Health Care and the Lessons for Britain*, London: Institute of Economic Affairs.

Green, D. (1987) *The New Right*, Brighton: Wheatsheaf.

Harris, R. (1988) *Beyond the Welfare State: An Economic, Political and Moral Critique of Indiscriminate State Welfare and a Review of Alternatives to Dependency*, London: Institute of Economic Affairs.

Hayek, F. (1960) *The Constitution of Liberty*, London: RKP.

Haywood, S. and Ranade, W. (1989) 'Privatising from within: the NHS under Thatcher', *Local Government Studies*, vol. 15, pp. 19–34.

Hindess, B. (1987) *Freedom, Equality and the Market*, London: Tavistock.

Honigsbaum, F., Richards, J. and Lockett, T. (1995) *Priority Setting for Health Care*, Oxford: Radcliffe Medical Press.

Jessop, B., Bonnett, K., Bromley, F. and Ling, T. (1988) *Thatcherism: A Tale of Two Nations*, Cambridge: Polity.

Joseph, K. and Sumption, J. (1979) *Equality*, London: John Murray.

Kendall, I. and Moon, G. (1990) 'Health Policy', in S. Savage and L. Robins (eds), *Public Policy under Thatcher*, London: Macmillan.

Kendall, I. and Moon, G. (1994) 'Health Policy and the Conservatives', in S. Savage, R. Atkinson and L. Robins (eds), *Public Policy in Britain*, London: Macmillan.

Klein, R. (1995) *The New Politics of the NHS*, London: Longman.

Marsland, D. (1988) 'The welfare state as a producer monopoly', *Salisbury Review*, vol. 6, pp. 4–9.

Ministry of Health (1956) *Report of the Committee of Enquiry into the Costs of the NHS*, Cmd 9663, London: HMSO.

Mohan, J. (1995) *A National Health Service?*, London: Macmillan.

Mooney, G. (1986) *Economics, Medicine and Health Care*, London: Harvester Wheatsheaf.

Niskanen, W. (1971) *Bureaucracy and Representative Government*, Chicago: Aldine.

Nozick, R. (1974) *Anarchy, State and Utopia*, Oxford: Blackwell.

OECD (1993) *OECD Health Systems: facts and trends 1960–91*, Paris: OECD.

Petchey, R. (1987) 'Health maintenance organisations: just what the doctor ordered?', *Journal of Social Policy*, vol. 16, pp. 489–509.

Powell, J. (1966) *Medicine and Politics*, London: Pitman.

Ranade, W. (1994) *A Future for the NHS?*, London: Longman.

Royal Commission on the NHS (1979) *Report of the Royal Commission on the NHS*, Cmnd 7615, London: HMSO.

Sackett, D., Haynes, R. and Tugwell, P. (1985) *Clinical Epidemiology: A Basic Science For Clinical Medicine*, Boston: Little Brown.

Scheffler, R. (1989) 'Adverse selection: the Achilles' heel of the NHS reforms', *Lancet*, vol. 99, pp. 950–52.

Secretary of State for Health (1989) *Working for Patients*, Cmnd 555, London: HMSO.

Stevens, A. and Gabbay, J. (1991) 'Needs assessment needs assessment', *Health Trends*, vol. 23, pp. 20–23.

Strong, P. and Robinson, J. (1990) *The NHS Under New Management*, Milton Keynes: Open University Press.

Tomlinson, B. (1992) *Report of the Inquiry into London's Health Service, Medical Education and Research*, London: HMSO.

Townsend, P., Davidson, N. and Whitehead, M. (1992) *Inequalities in Health*, Harmondsworth: Penguin.

Williams, A. (1978) ' "Need": an economic exegesis', in A. Culyer and K. Wright (eds), *Economic Aspects of Health Services*, London: Robertson.

7

Consumers, Service Users or Citizens?

Nancy North

As discussed in Chapter 1, the welfare state created in the post-war United Kingdom was sustained for the next twenty or so years by a political consensus. According to Kavanagh (1987) there was continuity not only in key policy principles, but also in the way in which policies were developed. In the National Health Service (NHS) this was reflected in a broad commitment to the founding principles, despite the increasing resources this required, and an unshaken belief in the value of the contribution that the medical profession could bring to decision making at all levels of the NHS. The role ascribed to the service user was passive, with little or no opportunity to exercise 'voice' in the planning of services or 'choice' over aspects of treatment. The NHS was a 'monument to enlightened paternalism' (Klein, 1984: 17).

During the 1970s this indulgent but controlling approach was challenged from a number of directions. From the New Right viewpoint, not only did the welfare state deny citizens the right to make personal choices about their welfare but the results of this paternalistic and bureaucratic process were unsatisfactory. Only individuals could make correct choices about the value of a welfare service to them. In addition to this liberalist argument, the New Right criticised the inefficiency and insensitivity of welfare bureaucracies, cushioned as they were by regular budgetary allocations of resources from largely unquestioning governments. One solution was to allow the individual to become a true consumer of welfare and utility services, exercising his/her role as citizen by monitoring the activities of local government and national state and by actions which contributed to the welfare of the local community in some way. Thus the rights and entitlements of citizens were framed in relation to a minimalist welfare state which 'freed' the citizen to make his/her own choices but which required in return a duty to behave responsibly. The privatisation of welfare services, including the NHS, was a logical step towards the realisation of this for many theorists (for example, Pirie and Butler, 1988). Politicians, however, have been more cautious, as well they might be, given the popularity of the NHS. A more moderate solution had to be found.

There were echoes of the New Right's criticisms in the political left's view of welfare bureaucracies as controlling, insensitive and ill-serving. Eschewing privatisation, though not a mixed economy of welfare and the choice this theoretically brings, they identified the need to decentralise and democratise services, encouraging a greater involvement in decision making and ensuring greater accountability. Support for greater responsiveness to service users also sprang from the growth of popular consumer awareness, which in health care was channelled into a variety of interest groups (Hambleton, 1989). Some of these groups presented a challenge to the ethos and practice of established professional groups.

Empowerment? Consumerism and Democracy

Before examining the approach of recent Conservative governments to consumerism and democracy within the NHS, it is worth examining the concepts in some detail. Consumers within private markets are endowed with a degree of power in that they have the money to make the purchase. It is assumed that in an ideal market providers will want to compete over quality and price; they will take note of the responses of consumers as exemplified either by demand patterns or by the more focused method of consumer surveys and reviews of complaints about products. Because of imbalances in power between providers and individual consumers in particular, most markets are regulated by laws which provide protection against monopolies and against consumer exploitation. Consumer law requires providers to give accurate information about the product and provides some form of redress for faulty goods. The regulation of monopolies reinforces competition and the ultimate sanction of the market, namely the power of exit or the ability to desert one provider for another.

This may work reasonably well with tins of beans but health – or rather health *care* – is a rather different matter. Medical information is complex and requires 'translation' by the practitioner, which puts the consumer at a disadvantage. Some patients may be unable to make decisions themselves and even the most assertive and articulate individual may be overwhelmed by the circumstances. This imbalance between consumer and 'provider' knowledge is supposedly compensated by a professional ethical code which celebrates the the primacy of a patient's well-being, a notion which cloaks the commodification of health care. Unsurprisingly other things apparently influence the 'supply' of health care. Calnan *et al.*, (1992) found a relationship between the method of payment – capitation or fee for service – and the amount of time doctors devoted to clinical practice. Where payment was linked to capitation, proportionately less time was spent on clinical activity. Where the cost of care is borne by a third party (employer or insurance company) there is no financial disincentive for the patient to reject treatment. In the USA, where fee-for-service payments prevailed, this propensity for self-indulgence on the part of professionals and patients led to the introduction of measures to control spiralling costs by both third party insurers and the Reagan and Bush administrations. This has resulted in consumers paying more at the point of treatment and having less choice of provider, particularly at the secondary care level. Nevertheless potential consumers in the USA still have wide choice of insurers and insurance packages which relate to different modes of provision. Surpassing all concerns about costs, however, is the problem of the medically indigent in largely privatised health care systems. Unable to enter health care markets on the basis of either private or state-subsidised insurance schemes, these non-consumers have to rely on stigmatised and restricted state or voluntary provision.

Despite the difficulties of privatised welfare markets, there are lessons to be learned for those who wish to strengthen the position of the client or service user in state welfare systems. Potter (1988) identifies a number of consumerist principles relevant to public sector services, which in some cases overlap with democratic approaches to health care planning. They are access, choice, information, redress and participation, which in its weakest form is taken to mean consultation. At first glance these might seem uncontroversial, but in the context of a collectively funded state health service strategic decisions about access, choice of treatment and perhaps who treats need to be made by those who are politically accountable. A balance has to be struck between individual needs, population needs and the broader obligation to society.

Democratic approaches represent an alternative means of empowerment. A basic requirement of democracies is that those who hold office and take decisions on behalf of others are accountable to them for their actions – representative democracy. The locus of political accountability is significant. In the UK central government is ultimately responsible for the NHS and takes all the major decisions about funding and strategic direction. Citizens in theory can register their approval or rejection of a basket of policies at the ballot box – a crude and distant mechanism at best. The inadequacies of a political system in which power and policy making is centralised are one reason for the support of political devolution and greater participation within social democratic approaches. They also identify the need for welfare rights to enable social participation, a necessary precursor to citizenship. As discussed in Chapter 1, neo-conservative elements within New Right doctrine conceive of citizens contributing to the community freely while neo-liberalism is critical of the burden of a state welfare programme supported by taxes. Where the state is forced to become involved in the welfare of its citizens, there is a reluctance to encourage political representation. Hambleton and Hoggett suggest that, 'for the New Right, representative democracy inherently tends towards bureaucratic administration' (1990: 20), something to be avoided at all costs. Conservative decentralisation strategies within the public sector thus focus on managerial and organisational systems, rather than political devolution. This is not to argue that the new public management is ideologically neutral; it is a powerful vehicle for the promulgation of cultural change within the NHS and other welfare state structures.

Democratic approaches can move beyond the principle of elected representatives accountable to their local population to something which embraces a community-wide involvement in health care. The World Health Organisation's declaration at Alma Ata endorsed community participation as the means by which 'individuals and families assume responsibility for their own health and for those of the community, and develop the capacity to contribute to their own and their community's development' (WHO, 1978: 20). This contrasts sharply with the insular and somewhat passive role of consumer. It requires of individuals duties as well as rights; the duty not only to contribute to the welfare of the community, but also to take responsibility for their own health. There are resonances with the Conservative's view of citizenship, but the WHO definition goes much further. Its conceptualisation of citizenship mirrors social democratic approaches in that the community is involved in the definition and prioritisation of health care needs and the planning of health care by way of formal and informal representation. Later in this chapter we will examine the extent to which the present-day NHS reflects this approach.

Consumerism and Democracy in the NHS before 1979

Consumerist initiatives within the NHS are closely associated with internal markets for which the government sets out a number of aims. Applying Potter's (1988) principles, the NHS before the reforms was in many respects a bleak habitat for the would-be consumer – 'the ghosts in the NHS machinery' (Klein, 1989: 77). Though access to primary care was good and secondary care in the NHS excelled in the treatment of urgent and dangerous ill health, patients awaiting hospital-based treatment with non-life threatening problems had to live up to their name. Waiting lists are one manifestation of rationing within health care systems in which resources are allocated by planning processes rather than the market; the market itself enforces rationing through price.

Choice of general practitioner (GP) existed but, despite increasing interest in general practice as a specialism in the 1970s and 1980s, pressure from within the profession to limit list size and the control of numbers entering the medical profession have not encouraged GPs to compete for patients. The process for changing GPs was bureaucratic and acted as a deterrent. In addition, discriminatory practices in medical school admissions until the early 1970s resulted in restricted numbers of women graduates entering medicine and little choice for those patients who might prefer to be seen by a woman. Furthermore there is evidence which suggests that black applicants to medical school (Esmail *et al.*, 1995) and applicants to hospital medical posts (Esmail and Everington, 1993) have been discriminated against. The conclusion to be drawn from this and other research is that there was and still is considerable racial discrimination in medicine (McKenzie, 1995), including general practice. This is an unsatisfactory state of affairs which also effectively limits choice for those patients who, for language or cultural reasons, might prefer to see a black GP.

Exercising choice was also a difficult process for patients. Other than in those cases where the patient had changed address, GPs had to give signed consent to the patient's request to change practice. Access to and choice of care at secondary and tertiary levels (general and specialist acute care facilities) depended, as it still does, on the GP's assessment, but a GP could in theory refer the patient to any hospital in the country. For information about treatment options, patients had to rely on the opinions of their GPs. Objective and understandable information about the practice, local hospitals and the quality of treatment was hard to come by. In part these difficulties inhere in the complexity of medical knowledge and judgements but in the NHS, unlike more privatised health care systems, decisions about treatments were not influenced by provider incentives to oversupply. In contrast, the problem for the majority of patients was more one of speedy access to secondary and tertiary care.

The creation of Community Health Councils (CHCs) in 1974 provided institutional representation for consumers. A third of members were chosen by local voluntary bodies representing client groups, half by local authorities and the remainder by regional health authorities. As Klein (1989) points out, their composition resulted in a degree of functional ambiguity for CHCs, related to whether their obligation lay with representing the interests of consumers or a broader constituency. They attempted to combine responsibilities such as helping individual patients chart their way through NHS complaints procedures with more strategic functions, such as commenting on health authorities' plans. CHCs were given few resources. They were dependent on health authorities for information and access to planning teams, an unsatisfactory arrangement given their responsibilities. Relationships with health authorities were not always constructive, with CHCs experiencing difficulties in gaining access to information (Levitt, 1980). Levitt also concluded that there was a tendency for CHCs to regard their own opinion as representative of the general public when in fact their constituency was much narrower. Ham's (1992) not dissimilar view is that they promoted the voice of consumer groups at both the local level and nationally through their representative body, the Association of Community Health Councils. CHCs, therefore, were not an emphatically democratic force within the NHS yet they reflected a model of consumerism which was collective in its approach. Unfortunately their power was limited (Hunter, 1980; Shultz and Harrison, 1983), characterised by Klein as 'the ability to throw grit into the normal machinery of NHS decision-making' (1989: 116).

If consumerism was not a strong entity before the NHS reforms, neither was democracy. Few would describe the NHS system of governance as an exemplar of popular participation. Although its structure was broken down geographically and by level, the resulting authorities were not representative bodies since their membership comprised professionals, lay individuals and local authority representatives who were appointed, not elected. Consideration of the possibility of making local authorities responsible for health care, thus institutionalising political accountability, was abandoned in anticipation of fierce opposition from the medical profession. Formal political accountability lay with government and, given this model, it might have been assumed that the local NHS would be responsive to policies initiated by the centre. However evidence suggests that some initiatives, such as the proposed shift of resources to community care from the mid-1970s onwards, were effectively sidelined. The diversion of resources from areas which traditionally had received the support of the medical establishment proved difficult (Haywood and Alaszewski, 1980; Ham, 1981). The profession's interests were represented on committees at regional, area (until 1982) and district level, but the concept of clinical autonomy (see Chapter 5) meant that clinical practices – which generated the demand for health care resources – went unchallenged. 'It was clinical doctors who decided which patients to accept, how to investigate and treat them, whether to admit them to hospital, and how long to keep them there' (Harrison and Pollitt, 1994: 35). Both formal and informal decision-making mechanisms – essentially professional networks – at the local level thus succeeded in isolating the NHS from political mandate.

Consumerism, Participation and Representation after 1979

The Conservatives swept into office with an agenda which, true to the New Right prescription, sought to 'roll back the state', thereby reducing public expenditure. Nationalised industries such as gas and electricity were floated on the stock market and welfare services were subjected to financial constraints. As well as fiscal control there was a determination to secure effectiveness in the NHS, responding to Sir Roy Griffiths' doubts about 'Whether the NHS is meeting the needs of the patient and the community, and can prove that it is doing so' (DHSS, 1983: 10). Griffiths endeavoured to promote the notion of health care in which, as well as defining managerial accountability, responsiveness to the service user was encouraged. In respect of the latter aim, proof of success in the years following the introduction of the Griffiths Report remains equivocal. Subsequent research by Pollitt *et al.* (1991) reveals a cynicism on the part of medical and nursing staff about the introduction of consumerist measures and a preoccupation of management with staying within budget.

In a staccato foreword to *Working for Patients* (DoH, 1989), Margaret Thatcher stated that the government's aim was to 'extend patient choice, delegate responsibility to where services are provided and to secure the best value for money' (1989: not paginated). As a policy instrument, *Working for Patients* emphatically promoted a consumerist rather than a democratic approach, predicated on the belief that an internal market would secure further efficiency gains and make the NHS more responsive to the needs of patients. The needs of the local population were to be defined and articulated by health authorities; GP fundholders would appraise and, if appropriate, purchase care for individual patients (see Chapter 6 for a more detailed discussion). Pursuing the private sector model, the arrangements for health authorities seemed like a further retreat from any semblance of democracy in the NHS. The reforms reduced the number of members to a maximum of 11, which included five executive officers. Formal representation of the professions was eliminated, local authorities could no longer nominate representatives and Community Health Councils lost their speaking rights. Family Practitioner Committees (FPC) retained formal professional representations but professionals were in a minority in the reduced membership. The new-style authorities were modelled on private sector boards of directors and the recruitment process which followed encouraged applications from people with experience in business (Ashburner and Cairncross, 1993). As before, non-executive members were appointed, not elected. Health authorities, which since April 1996 incorporate the former FPC functions, theoretically have the power to make decisions about service models unfettered by historic patterns which combined demand and supply in the same institution. However these new freedoms are counterbalanced by a framework of priorities instituted by the centre and enforced by means of an effective managerial culture. *Working for Patients* implicitly recognises this: 'The overall effect of these changes will be to introduce for the first time a clear and effective chain of management command running from Districts through to Regions to the Chief Executive and from there to the Secretary of State' (DoH, 1989: 16).

Borrowing Hambleton's (1989) discriminating concepts, the reforms constituted an administrative rather than a political decentralisation. Fundamental decisions which affect the overall direction of the NHS remain the prerogative of the centre. Decentralisation of political power in the NHS would have meant the creation of locally accountable health authorities with an elected membership. Alternatively the UK could have followed the example of Sweden, where control over the provision of health services exists at county or municipal level and where, coincidentally, the system gives consumers greater choice (Saltman, 1994).

The membership of the new authorities was designed to complement the restructuring of the NHS to form an internal market in which the purchasers are either the Health Commission or GP fundholding practices. There were two basic concessions extended to consumers. The first related to tax relief on private insurance premiums for those aged 60 or over. The Treasury were no doubt mollified by the knowledge that this measure would entice a section of the population for whom it is costly to provide health care to exit from the NHS for some treatment. The second concession was to introduce a simpler procedure for changing GPs, in other words facilitating the power of exit from one primary health care provider to another. GPs were encouraged to try and retain patients by the restructuring of their payments. Capitation fees, paid for each patient on a GP's list, were to be increased so that this would contribute a greater proportion of the GP's income. The crude psychology underlying these changes was that GPs would work all the harder to attract patients to their practices.

The success of these initiatives is open to question. The Conservative government conceded that the tax concessions for elderly patients had not proved popular, an unsurprising outcome given that private insurance policies for elderly clients are expensive propositions. In addition there is little evidence to suggest that patients are changing

GPs more readily. Past studies indicate a high level of satisfaction with GP services (Williams and Calnan, 1991; Judge and Solomon, 1993) and the security afforded by familiarity plus the disincentive of travelling greater distances discourage change. In contrast to patient selectivity, there are reports that GPs are deregistering patients from their practices more frequently (*Sunday Times*, 16 October 1994). This suggests something more than GPs exercising their traditional right to rid themselves of difficult or abusive patients. Future research may well show a reduced tolerance level and a redefining of the problem patient such that practice boundaries are redrawn to exclude the more distant patients or whole 'problem estates'. Provider power still dominates in general practice.

The force of consumerist approaches within the NHS and Community Care Act 1990 lay in the creation of proxy consumers. GP fundholders and health authorities took on the role of health care purchasers. Both health authorities and providers have undertaken a considerable range of consumer consultation and consumer feedback exercises. In both these cases this work might effectively be seen as market research, the primary aim being to ensure that appropriate service packages were being purchased and that the quality of service provision was acceptable. The Patient's Charter (DoH, 1991) exacerbated this process by creating standards by which the health care consumer could assess the performance of a provider facility. In addition, the publication of indicators which compared hospital performances was specifically designed to provide the public with information about which hospitals were 'better'. Nevertheless it was about information for the market rather than consumer empowerment (Moon and Lupton, 1995). The decision about where patients went for treatment lay with the purchasers.

The organisational split between purchasers and providers brings with it the potential to shift resources from services whose budgets in the past reflected unchallenged medical practices which were protected by precedent and medical syndicalism. In 1996 the statutory fusion of DHAs and Family Health Service Authorities (who supervise general practitioner services, dental services and community pharmacists) created health authorities with a strategic overview of all health services and integrated commissioning. In many areas this was anticipated with the development of functioning 'shadow' authorities. The task of health authorities can be summarised thus: identifying the health needs of their local population, prioritising those needs, deciding which treatment approaches, service models and providers offer the most cost-effective option and purchasing services accordingly.

This is a complex undertaking which in the needs assessment phase relies in part on epidemiological, clinical effectiveness and cost effectiveness data, but also on the opinions of health professionals and, in theory, the wider population. As such it seeks to blend rational–scientific and political approaches to decision making. Market dynamics are excluded, but the market nevertheless endows certain of the participants with influence over the process. The role of GPs and fundholders, in particular, is likely to be significant. There are steadily increasing numbers of GP fundholders boosted by a new initiative creating additional categories of fundholding which became operational in April 1996. Although health authorities retain important purchasing responsibilities, including contracting health care on behalf of patients of non-fundholding practices, high cost care and the more specialised services, the growth in fundholding will result in a recasting of their role (North, 1995).

By weakening the power of consultants, the reforms opened up the possibility of more pluralistic decision making – local issue networks taking the place of closed policy networks in health authorities. Amid the flurry of working papers and guidelines issued after the 1990 NHS and Community Care Act, *Local Voices* (NHSME, 1992) focused on health authorities'/commission's responsibilities to consult local people. It exhorts health authorities to develop 'a champion of the people role' which would 'enhance the credibility of health authorities' and be more likely to result in services 'better suited to local needs' (1992: 3). This advice conflates representational and consumerist approaches. At heart it seems to be about legitimising the activities of health authorities. The guidelines go on to discuss the involvement of local people in priority setting and the development and monitoring of services is to be achieved through the processes of information giving, discussion, consultation and participation, an approach which seems to glide beyond consumerism into a more democratic, WHO-type model of participative decision making involving the community – something more akin to Lindblom's pluralistic notion of partisan mutual adjustment.

Set against this apparently more open approach to consultation and participation, the more restricted role for CHCs seems anomalous. Their speaking rights on health authorities were removed and trusts were allowed to decide for themselves whether to allow CHCs access to routine meetings. CHCs can still inspect local providers, but only within the district. The development of cross-boundary contracting will therefore limit their effectiveness unless they can exchange views with neighbouring CHCs. The designation of purchasers as 'champions of the people' and the inevitable focusing of provider attention on Patient's Charter standards and hospital performance league table have cast a shadow over the continuing role of CHCs.

Problems and Possibilities

Health authorities remain firmly in charge of a process which purports to solicit the views of more stakeholders than formerly. The task is far from simple. While other stakeholders, such as providers or GPs, are clearly defined, the requirement to consult local people raises problems of whom to consult over which issues and the method of consultation used. Service user groups are well informed about the particular needs of those they represent and can contribute much in consultation exercises about service models and treatment outcomes, whereas the woman in the street cannot. Service user groups can also raise concerns about unmet needs, which should be fed into discussions about the prioritisation of particular health problems and the overall allocation of resources. The increasing involvement of these groups in service provision, characteristically in the area of long-term community rehabilitation and support, raises the question of whether they can offer impartial advice, isolated from any 'provider agendas'. The same could be said of the role of professional expertise in contributing to needs assessments. Given the finite finances of the NHS, the success of one group in getting its needs met imposes a cost on other service users. The prioritisation of needs is therefore important and demands a more democratic process and a broader constituency than user – or professional – groups alone.

Information giving and consultation both figure among Potter's (1988) principles of consumerism and are advocated in *Local Voices*. It suggests that information should be easily understood and adequate to support locally informed debate. There lies a difficulty: the process of distilling highly complex information about clinical effectiveness, treatment costs and health gain measurements relating to debates about priorities is not itself value-free. Attempts to simplify information risks distortion. There is the ever-present danger of manipulation, a whisker away from the suggestion in *Local Voices* that health authorities are likely to exert more leverage on providers 'if they secure public support' (1992: 3) for difficult decisions. It is perhaps as important to expose the underlying rationale and processes leading to published information so that others may challenge conclusions. This is an argument for better information as opposed to simply more.

Consultation processes could influence commissioning but the values underlying the process are critical. Harrison and Wistow (1992) found diverse approaches to public consultation among health authorities. Surveys may reach large numbers of service users and/or the lay public, but they can be constructed so that options are limited or, worse still, responses manipulated to produce the desired result (Coote, 1993). The most critical question of all, whether individuals would pay a hypothecated tax to increase funding to the NHS, is absent from the contemporary political agenda.

The encouragement to health authorities to consult widely is laudable and there is early evidence of attempts to reach those sections of the population whose voice has been rarely heard in the past. Preliminary findings of a DoH-commissioned survey on the efforts of purchasers and providers to 'deal with issues of ethnic minority health' indicated there were a number of current initiatives which involved 'researching health needs, hearing "local voices" and developing culturally sensitive services' (NHSE and The Kings Fund, 1995: 1). According to the respondents (health authorities and providers), strategies for consultation included focus and user groups and 'consumer conferences' (ibid.). Minority groups were consulted over specific issues as well as being involved in formal planning cycles and the prioritisation of purchasing options.

Though improving on the restricted consultation processes of the past, such arrangements are not about surrendering decision making to a wider forum. Health authorities are reminded that local views may have to be overridden 'on the weight of epidemiological, resource or other considerations' (NHSME, 1992: 3). Consultation with service users, local community groups or broader-based surveys of local opinion thus forms a part of a much larger information-gathering process which involves other interested parties listed by

Local Voices as GPs, providers and local authorities, local politicians and the media. It is the task of the health authority/commission managers to evaluate and blend all the information to produce policy options which the health authority/commission members then decide on. The encouragement that *Local Voices* gave to a more pluralistic consultation process may well be overshadowed by other developments. The National Health Service Executive, anticipating a growth in fundholding, encouraged health authorities to orchestrate the contribution of GPs to strategic development (EL(94)79) (NHSE, 1994). This is a pragmatic move, since needs assessment is a far from perfect science (Stevens and Gabbay, 1992) and thus requires a political means of legitimation. If fundholding continues after the election scheduled in 1997, the purchasing power of fundholders will accord them an inevitable and increasing influence on the local policy-making process. The reforms will have replaced one institutionalised form of medical power with another.

Consultation with the public or with service users, as promoted in *Local Voices*, does not guarantee influence over policy making, but then this would not be without danger. In addition to the need to strike a balance between the preferences of clients and those of the wider population, Klein (1984) identifies a further difficulty: consumer preferences reflect knowledge of what is available rather than what is possible, and are biased towards the acute services. This latter observation was confirmed by Bowling *et al.*'s (1993) research in which the general public prioritised neonatal intensive care rather than care for schizophrenic patients. If this populist tendency were to be repeated across the breadth of commissioning, 'minority' services, or those which do not receive media attention, such as psychogeriatric services, would be shunted to the end of the queue. So too might the needs of ethnic minorities. It is in the nature of democracies to marginalise minority views. The fact that complex health decisions about resource allocation between health needs should not be made on the basis of a popularity poll is an argument not only for informed decision making by selected, accountable representatives, but also for better education of the general public about the issues. It also calls for iterative processes which inform and enable dialogue rather than the 'quick-fix' use of surveys.

It might appear less problematic to consult the views of the public or service users on specific services and therapies rather than priorities, although again the pairing of constituency and issue is important. Most people would be able to suggest improvements they would wish to see in general practice despite not holding an opinion on specialised care services. There is more of a problem in getting active service users to criticise the services on offer, a tendency observed by Wilson (1993) in her research on community health and social services. Saltman (1994) notes similarities between the halo effect and the 'Stockhom Syndrome' where the behaviour of hostages during a bank siege demonstrated that they had identified with the needs of their captors. Though this is rather an extreme analogy, it should not be forgotten that clients are often in a position of vulnerability and dependent on the disposition of professionals for treatment and support. These observations suggest that in-house consumer surveys by providers are likely to be seriously flawed, even if the legitimate question of a vested interest on the part of providers is ignored. If information gathering for service development or the evaluation of services is to be undertaken at all, it may be more appropriate to fund Community Health Councils.

Undiscriminating gratitude on the part of the public relates more widely to the problem of securing *informed* opinion. Shoddy service in a restaurant or a poor product in a supermarket is not too difficult to recognise, but the same cannot be said for health care. To a limited degree the Patient's Charter attempted to improve the situation by publishing 'three new rights': to be given information about local health services, to be guaranteed a period no longer than two years on a hospital waiting list and to receive a prompt and written response to any complaint about NHS services. The Charter also established nine standards which ranged from the fairly vague requirement that, subject to his/her wishes, relatives be kept informed of a patient's progress, to the more precise admonishment that outpatient clinics forswear the practice of booking in several patients to see a consultant at the same time. As from 1 April 1992, individual appointment times were to be given and patients could expect to be seen within 30 minutes of that time. Other standards, however, were disappointing. After presumably being kept on an admissions waiting list for up to two years, a patient could have their operation postponed twice before receiving an alternative date within one month of the final postponement. In most European countries and the USA this would be considered a very poor state of affairs indeed.

The changing ethos of the NHS and the reconstitution of patients as consumers has added an additional urgency to the much needed reform of a complex complaints system. In May 1994, the Wilson committee produced its review of the NHS complaints procedure. *Being Heard* observed that the existing arrangements presented many hurdles to the would-be complainant. The means by which complaints could be registered were obscure and there were too many different procedures across the health service. Complainants were often left feeling frustrated by the process and dissatisfied with the outcome. The report recommended changes based on three principles: there should be a common complaints system covering all NHS services, including general practice; the complaints system should be kept separate from disciplinary processes and be geared to the complainant's concerns; there should be a two-stage approach: an in-house review of the complaint and, if this fails, an investigation by an independent panel. Emphasis was placed on dealing with the complaint as swiftly as possible, preferably by staff at hand. The committee also called for support of complainants and respondents, acknowledging the stress placed on both parties. The report provides a much needed appraisal of the hitherto defensive arrangements. There is a sense that the recommendations are welcome, not only for the more straightforward and humane approach they bring to complaints procedure, but also because they may cope better with the increased number of complaints. In England, the number of complaints made to hospital and community trusts has risen dramatically. In the year 1993/4 this figure represented a 330 per cent increase on the number of complaints in 1983, with the rate of increase accelerating year by year (source of data: DoH, 1995).

Whether the levels of dissatisfaction this registers arise from the inability of an inadequately resourced health service to meet the needs of individuals or the raised expectations of a consumer-minded clientele, or a combination of the two, is difficult to ascertain. In the changed culture of the NHS, mirroring as it does the world of commerce, the possibility of friction between provider and recipient of care is greater. Failure will be all the more obvious because stated objectives have not been met (Jacobs, 1991). In the short term individual patients or their lawyers are less likely to be in possession of meaningful standards by which they can successfully prosecute a complaint, but the growth of audit makes medical practice increasingly susceptible to litigation. Legal redress, or threat of it, is perhaps the ultimate mechanism of exerting consumer power and represents a nightmare scenario for health authorities and professionals alike.

Summary

In Chapter 2 of this book we examined various explanations of the policy process, raising the deceptively simple question, 'Who has the power?' Various chapters have identified the determination of the New Right to excise exclusionary, professional arrangements in the welfare state which, it was claimed, not only inflated the supply of services over what was required but fashioned services according to the views of professional elites. The solution in the case of the NHS and other welfare services was to introduce a quasi-market. On the face of it this organisational transformation, by ending previous routines of resource allocation, limited the influence of professionals in the provider units. The medical profession's claim to represent the interests of clients has been superseded by the notion that health authorities represent and balance the interests of the local population. This role is most clearly evident in the process of needs assessment and prioritisation whereby the contributions of service users and/or other conceptualisations of 'local people' are actively sought (Pickard *et al.*, 1995).

To this extent, influence in local policy making might be described as more pluralistic; it does not imply that the power of all the stakeholders – professionals, local people, other agencies and GPs – is equal. In the words of one senior health commission manager, 'those with the power are those with the money' – in other words health authorities and GP fundholders (North, unpublished thesis). Tacit recognition of the power of purchasers means that, if fund-holding survives the next election, not only will fundholders be drawn increasingly into needs assessment and the development of purchasing strategies, but they will have the final say on what is purchased. Nor can the influence of other doctors be ignored; in the absence of robust scientific information on the effectiveness of treatments let alone more complex, 'organic' service models which rely on multi-disciplinary co-operation, the opinions of experts still have strong currency.

Paradoxically some form of consultation remains the strongest hope for health service users. New Right support for a more active role for consumers in education could not be duplicated in health care. Demand for education is a function of the numbers of schoolchildren in the system; demand for health care is potentially infinite. Margaret

Thatcher's government avoided radical and politically suicidal options in refashioning the health service and instead chose an attenuated form of consumerism: individuals are only permitted to express consumer choice in the selection of their GP or discontent via the complaints system. The emphasis on providing better services may promote dissatisfaction as expectations are not realised. Although in Glennerster *et al.*'s (1994) study many GP fundholders expressed a belief that their purchasing power would bring improved care for their patients, this is quite different from allowing patients a choice of several treatments or providers, or involving them in purchasing decisions. A great deal will depend on the ability of health authorities to identify and incorporate local patient groups in formal decision-making processes.

Even so, it is too early to say whether the broader consultation process will result in radical change. The policy of community care for people with mental health and learning difficulties and the trend towards shorter periods of hospitalisation for other patient groups may well meet resistance from both GPs and groups where carers form a powerful element of the membership who bear the brunt of any inadequate resourcing. Opportunistic coalitions such as this may represent the best way forward for local 'consumer' groups who may lack both experience and influence. Effective opposition would, ironically, mean that community care policies might prove as difficult to implement at the local level as they were before the reforms to health and social care services.

The lack of empirical evidence to support an analysis of patient or consumer power in the NHS compounds an already difficult debate. Perhaps the major difference the reforms have made is the most insidious and difficult to estimate in both its extent and effect. The dominant values and culture of the NHS emphasise efficiency and effectiveness in meeting the needs of the local population. The real hope for patients, carers and the well is that these terms are not so narrowly defined as to exclude lay knowledge. If that were to happen there is more likelihood of community agendas being marginalised and purchasing decisions reflecting an accommodation between medical and managerial experts. In the absence of effective consumer (as opposed to agency purchaser) power in the NHS, consultation and representation which is locally accountable seem to be legitimate ways forward.

Bibliography

Ashburner, L. and Cairncross, L. (1993) 'Membership on the "New Style" Health Authorities: Continuity or Change?', *Public Administration*, vol. 71, Autumn, pp. 357–75.

Bowling, A., Jacobson, B. and Southgate, L. (1993) 'Explorations in consultation of the public and health professionals on priority setting in an inner London health district', *Social Science and Medicine*, vol. 37, no. 7, pp. 851–7.

Calnan, M., Groenewegen, P. P. and Hutten, J. (1992) 'Professional reimbursement and management of time in general practice', *Social Science and Medicine*, vol. 35, no. 12, pp. 209–16.

Coote, A. (1993) Public Participation in decisions about health care, *Critical Public Health*, vol. 4, no. 1, pp. 36–48.

DHSS (1983) *NHS Management Inquiry* (The Griffiths Report), London: DHSS.

DoH (1989) *Working for Patients* Cmnd 555, London: HMSO.

DoH (1991) *The Patient's Charter*, London: HMSO.

DoH (1995) *Written Complaints by or on behalf of patients, England, Financial Year 1993–94*, Government Statistical Service, London: Department of Health.

Esmail, A, Nelson, P., Primarolo, D., Toma, T. (1995) 'Acceptance into medical school and racial discrimination', *British Medical Journal*, vol. 310, pp. 501–2.

Esmail, A. and Everington, S. (1993) 'Racial discrimination against doctors from ethinic minorities', *British Medical Journal*, vol. 306, pp. 691–2.

Glennerster, H., Matsanganis, M., and Owens, P. with Hancock, S. (1994) *Implementing GP Fundholding*, Buckingham: Open University Press.

Ham, C.J. (1981) *Policy Making in the National Health Service*, London: Macmillan.

Ham, C.J. (1992) *Health Policy in Britain*, 3rd edn, London: Macmillan.

Hambleton, R. (1989) 'Consumerism, decentralisation and local democracy', *Public Administration*, vol. 66, pp. 125–47.

Hambleton, R. (1992) 'Decentralisation and democracy in UK local government', *Public Money and Management*, July/September, pp. 9–20.

Hambleton, R. and Hoggett, P. (1990) *Beyond Excellence: Quality Local Government in the 1990s*, Working Paper 85, Bristol: S.A.U.S.

Harrison, S. and Pollitt, C. (1994) *Controlling Health Professionals. The future of work and organization in the NHS*, Buckingham: Open University Press.

Harrison, S. and Wistow, G. (1992) 'The purchaser/provider split in English health care: towards explicit rationing?' *Policy and Politics*, vol. 20, no. 2, pp. 123–30.

Haywood, S. and Alaszewski, A. (1980) *Crisis in the Health Service*, London: Croom Helm.

Hunter, D.J. (1980) *Coping with Uncertainty, Politics and Policy in the NHS*, Chichester: Research Studies Press.

Jacobs. J.M. (1991) 'Lawyers go to hospital', *Public Law*, Summer, pp. 255–81.

Judge, K. and Solomon, M. (1993) 'Patient Opinion and the National Health Service: Patterns and Perspectives', *Journal of Social Policy*, vol. 22, no. 3, pp. 299–327.

Kavanagh, D. (1987) *Thatcherism and British Politics*, Oxford: Clarendon Press.

Klein, R. (1984) 'The politics of participation', in R.J. Maxwell and N. Weaver (eds), *Public Participation in Health*, London: King Edward's Hospital Fund for London.

Klein, R. (1989) *The Politics of the NHS*, 2nd edn, London: Longman

Levitt, R. (1980) *The People's Voice in the NHS*, London: King Edward's Hospital Fund for London.

McKenzie, K.J. (1995) 'Racial discimination in medicine', *British Medical Journal*, vol. 310, pp. 478–9.

Moon, G. and Lupton, C. (1995) 'Within acceptable limits: health care provider perspectives on community health councils in the reformed National Health Service', *Policy and Politics*, vol. 23, pp. 335–46.

NHSE (1994) Developing NHS Purchasing and GP Fundholding: Towards a Primary Care-led NHS, Leeds: NHSE.

NHSE and the Kings Fund (1995) *Improving the Health of Ethnic Minority Communities*, Bulletin 4, Purchasing Innovations, April, Leeds: NHSE.

NHSME (1992) *Local Voices. The Views of Local People in Purchasing for Health*, London: DoH.

North, N. (1995) 'GP fundholding in 2000: David, Goliath or just history?' *Critical Public Health*, vol. 6, no. 1, pp. 11–19.

North, N. (1996) Commissioning Health Care in the NHS: A Study of the Process in one District Health Authority, (unpublished thesis) University of London.

Pickard, S., Williams, G. and Flynn, R. (1995) 'Local Voices in an Internal Market: the case of community health services', *Social Policy and Administration*, vol. 29, no. 2, pp. 135–49.

Pirie, M. and Butler, E. (1988) *The Health of Nations*, London: Adam Smith Institute.

Pollitt, C., Harrison, S., Hunter, D.J. and Marnoch, G. (1991) 'General Management in the NHS: the initial impact 1983–88', *Public Administration*, vol. 69, Spring, pp. 61–83.

Potter, J. (1988) 'Consumerism and the Public Sector: How well does the coat fit?' *Public Administration*, vol. 66, Summer, pp. 149–64.

Saltman, R.B. (1994) 'Patient choice and patient empowerment in Northern European health systems: a conceptual framework', *International Journal of Health Services*, vol. 24, no. 2, pp. 201–29.

Shultz, R. and Harrision, A. (1983) *Teams and Top Managers in the NHS: a survey and a strategy*, Project Paper No. 41, London: King's Fund.

Stevens, A. and Gabbay, J. (1991) 'Needs assessment needs assessment', *Health Trends*, vol. 23, pp. 20–23.

WHO (1978) *Alma Alta 1977. Primary Health Care*, Geneva: WHO, UNICEF.

Williams, S. and Calnan, M. (1991) 'Key determinants of consumer satisfaction with general practice', *Family Practice*, vol. 8, no. 3, pp. 237–42.

Wilson, G. (1993) 'Users and Providers: Different perspectives on community care services', *Journal of Social Policy*, vol. 22, no. 4, pp. 507–26.

8

Market Testing/Market Failure

Health Service Privatisation in Theory and Practice, 1979–96

John Mohan

Introduction

Writing in triumphalist vein at the height of the mid-1980s economic boom, John Redwood (1988) claimed that privatisation represented the most important economic phenomenon of the 1980s; he portrayed it as a global movement, sweeping all before it. However such a description was not only inaccurate with regard to the British welfare state (there were clearly some areas where the private sector's writ did not run), it also represented a limited and partial explanation of moves towards privatisation. For to present privatisation merely as a sweeping global phenomenon is to neglect its intellectual and political origins in specific national contexts, and subsumes a range of different types of, and rationales for, privatisation. Moreover it ignores the extent to which privatisation has – or has not – achieved its declared aims. Clearly it has gone further in some sectors than others. Redwood's views also neglect roads not taken: a triumphalist account such as his ignores the ways certain options were ruled off the political agenda and also ignores differences of opinion within the government of the day. It is therefore necessary to consider the attractions of and limits to privatisation.

Definitional points are also in order. In a narrow sense privatisation could be said to refer solely to the transfer of functions formerly

150

carried out by the state to the private sector. However, as the time-honoured typology of Le Grand and Robinson (1984) makes clear, the boundary between public and private goes beyond direct provision to encompass subsidy and regulation. More generally, it is at least arguable that there is a cultural dimension to privatisation, which is symbolised by the conflicts between individual and collective interests described in this chapter: privatisation has perhaps led to a shift in the attitudes and values of individuals and organisations within the NHS, such that the capture of benefits for private gain is seen as a legitimate form of behaviour. In addition privatisation has an important ideological content: its expansion possibly creates conditions in which people prioritise individualist rather than collective solutions, in which they seek to exit from collective provision. These two elements may be of more lasting significance than the direct fiscal or efficiency effects of privatisation.

Bearing these remarks in mind, this chapter is divided into three sections. The first considers privatisation in theory, looking at the rationales for it and some of the explanations which have been advanced for it. The second considers the development of privatisation in practice, documenting the principal elements of privatisation policies from 1979 and drawing out some key themes; this includes discussion of the limits to privatisation: in other words, the constraints on extending it beyond a quite limited proportion of health service activity. The concluding section evaluates the likely future of privatisation and whether it is consistent with a comprehensive, national health service.

Motivations for Privatisation

At least three sets of motivations for privatisation may be distinguished. Firstly, there are those who see privatisation as the natural outcome of processes operating in the economy and polity, and which impinge on all areas of the welfare state. From this perspective, just as states were formerly converging towards state provision of welfare services, they are now heading in the direction of a more pluralist model, in which the state may well remain the dominant partner, but in which community and commercial sources of care play an increasingly prominent role. Linked to this are arguments which suggest that levels of economic prosperity have produced a more discerning citizenry, who exercise choice in so many areas of social life that an extension of consumerism and choice into the welfare state is only natural. Such people are said to be accustomed to building up packages of welfare provision from a range of sources: commercial insurance is one obvious such source, although much of the growth in this has been led by company-paid schemes; the rise of alternative therapies is another (Sharma, 1991; Klein and Millar, 1995). From these perspectives, then, privatisation is a natural outcome of economic growth and of the growing emphasis on consumption as a form of social division and stratification (on which see Busfield, 1990).

Such arguments have not been unchallenged. Mishra (1990), for instance, sees in welfare pluralism a covert strategy for reductions in state provision, arguing that other sectors (commercial, charitable, the family) have 'not picked up the tab' when government has withdrawn from provision of services (see also Johnson, 1989). More crucially for our argument, welfare pluralism does not emerge from nowhere; it develops in a context – particularly so in the UK, where the state's role in providing and financing health care is arguably exceptional (OECD, 1993) – heavily structured by state decisions. It follows that a fuller understanding of privatisation is more likely to be found in the political realm. In this context we should differentiate between political philosophy and political strategy. Whatever the philosophical attractions of privatisation, the extent to which they could be realised in practice depended heavily on political constraints; moreover the Conservatives' economic and political programme during the 1980s arguably had several distinguishing characteristics, which points to the need for a contextualised account of the privatisation process.

In philosophical terms the most cogent arguments for privatisation – or, more accurately, against state intervention – were advanced by Hayek (for example, 1944), for whom state intervention, other than in a minimalist sense of protecting property rights, securing law and order, and national defence, was always repressive. More detailed planning and regulation threatened a moral order of individual responsibility, and was viewed by Hayek as ultimately coercive. Thus nationalisation is said to have stifled a whole range of community-based initiatives in health care which were said to be flourishing prior to the Second World War. Some have drawn on this to imply that the effect of the NHS was therefore to restrict choice below the level individuals would have freely chosen for themselves. Furthermore the state can never possess the intelligence required to co-ordinate markets effectively; the price mechanism reflects changes in demands, technologies and resources more quickly and effectively than the state ever could, and so markets reduce inflexibilities and promote more efficient allocation of resources. State agencies also develop interests in their own survival, and consequently they have been characterised as 'producer monopolies' (Marsland, 1988). In contrast, markets are proclaimed to be egalitarian and democratic: egalitarian because competition will in theory whittle away supranormal profits and therefore restrain costs; and democratic because markets enfranchise individuals rather than bureaucracies, and thus tailor services to individual needs. These arguments have been used to argue for a much greater degree of market control within the health service; if the purer versions of free-market ideology (such as insurance-based or voucher schemes) have been ruled out, competition has nevertheless been introduced in various guises.

However, even in theory, there are some objections to these views. Markets do not clear at the point at which all demand is met, so they are arguably incompatible with a comprehensive service. The decentralisation associated with markets raises questions about appropriate forms of regulation, to ensure the proper control of public money. Furthermore the fixed investment in health care institutions renders them highly inflexible, which raises questions about the ease with which they can adjust in response to market forces. In practice, moreover, it is questionable whether reliance on market forces will guarantee a comprehensive system. A careful examination of the pre-NHS hospital system, for instance, amply demonstrates the limitations to voluntarism (Webster, 1995; Powell, 1992), in contrast to the optimistic assertions of, for instance, Green (1994). Nor has the expansion of the commercial hospital sector in the UK been without difficulties, and so far coverage of the population is only 11 per cent, suggesting some clear limitations to reliance on market forces. There are clear theoretical and practical objections to the Hayekian blue print, though this is not to deny the influence that Hayek's thought has had on the Conservative government.

Rather than entailing the adoption of a theoretical blueprint, then, privatisation post-1979 has been marked by pragmatism and tactical advances and retreats. The kinds of privatisation proposed and implemented defy any attempt to impose a unitary interpretation; the particular motivations varied according to the issue in question.

Broadly speaking, however, one can see a range of initiatives as conforming with a political strategy designed selectively to promote the interests of key social strata and geographical locations. This has been described as a 'two nations' political project (Jessop *et al.*, 1987; 1988), working through a series of oppositions: private versus public, 'South' versus 'North', services versus manufacturing, 'independence' versus 'dependence', and so on. This was a multifaceted strategy and several strands may be drawn out of it. Firstly, the Conservatives clearly saw in the NHS various opportunities for recommodifying areas of activity which had been taken over by the state. From this perspective, competitive tendering was promoted as a means of stimulating small business formation and increasing flexibility within the service. There were multiple motivations for this: the public sector was demonised, during the 1978–9 winter of discontent, as the preserve of producer interests, to the detriment of consumers; it was also seen as being insulated from competitive labour market conditions. Breaking down national systems of labour regulation would therefore serve important ideological purposes, as well as releasing some funds to minimise pressure for increased government spending (although the extent of savings was always disputed). The abrogation of various forms of protection for workers was therefore an integral part of competitive tendering and the effect was a greater degree of fragmentation and division within the workforce.

Privatisation was also promoted through an ideological emphasis on self-help and a rhetorical stress on 'independence' rather than the dependency culture of the welfare state. Various forms of encouragement to the private sector were offered; although arguably these did not add up to very much, their contribution to the ideological climate was substantial in that they served to underline governmental messages about freedom of choice. Self-help was also stressed – notably an emphasis on the importance of the family and community as first ports of call, but also expanding scope for charitable and other forms of fund raising – while the consistent message was that the state's resources were finite, so that localist solutions were necessary to supplement public funds. Indeed at one point Patrick Jenkin, the Conservatives' first Secretary of State for Social Services, went so far as to argue that the NHS should best be seen as a collection of 'local' services rather than a national organisation. However his localist, pro-voluntarist stance was severely criticised for making heroic assumptions about the availability of resources in the community.

Finally it was argued, at first implicitly and later through explicit legislation, that the role of health authorities should be redefined, from being a monopoly provider of services to having an essentially 'coordinative, entrepreneurial role' (Davies, 1987); clearly, local capacities and resources were to play a greater role in the NHS than hitherto. We return to this tension between national and local later in this chapter.

Thus no single and consistent thread runs through these diverse changes. One sees in Conservative ideology a range of different motivations for change; some drew clearly upon the precepts of the New Right, while others were more inchoate, representing wishful anti-statism rather than coherent strategy (Wistow, 1988). As a consequence, the history of privatisation initiatives can be written as a series of experiments in market testing, in preparing the ground for possibly more far-reaching change.

Market Testing: the Extent of Efforts at Privatisation, 1979–96

The range of developments which could be held to constitute privatisation is considerable: Table 8.1 summarises the main features of these since 1979. This draws on Le Grand and Robinson's (1984) typology and seeks to show how the boundaries between public and private provision have shifted. Although many of the elements of this table are presented as being analytically separate, this cannot be sustained in practice: thus the expansion of private nursing homes cannot be separated from the changes to regulations which enabled those admitted to private long-stay nursing homes to claim support from the social security budget. As well as the more obvious attempts to shift the boundary between public and private spheres – encouraging private acute health care and expanding the scope for links between the public and private sectors being just two – there have been measures designed to enhance the extent to which services still under the direct supervision of the NHS operate on de facto commercial lines (competitive tendering) and more generally to expand the resource base on which the NHS draws beyond that of direct taxation (in the latter case, the proportion of NHS finance raised from direct taxation has been at an historic low while the contribution of other sources of income, notably land sales, has risen dramatically). Many initiatives essentially represent cost-shifting exercises, which pass the burden of finance or of care onto individuals and their families; though often hidden, such cost shifting really ought to be recorded somewhere in the balance sheet. Even measures designed to enhance efficiency and throughput within the NHS have the effect of shifting some of the burden of post-operative care onto patients' families. A vast range of initiatives have been undertaken and their full description is beyond the scope of this chapter. Instead it concentrates on the evolution of privatisation initiatives and some of the main themes therein.

A pure neo-liberal approach to health care policy would presumably involve an insurance-based system in which there was a direct connection between an individual's labour market position and access to health care. However there are technical obstacles to such systems, as the experience of the USA demonstrates, notably labour market inflexibilities: individuals are reluctant to change jobs for fear of losing health benefits (Besley and Gouveia, 1994). This is to say nothing of the likely political controversies. Consequently, on returning to office in 1979, the Conservatives made no immediate attempts to replace the NHS and indeed their manifesto commitments said relatively little other than their desire to expand the private sector. However the possibilities for alternatives to tax-based finance were explored, outside Government, by Conservative think tanks and, most famously, within government, by the Central Policy Review Staff (CPRS). The CPRS reported in late 1982 on the implications of a move towards an insurance-based system and their report was leaked, causing considerable controversy. Reports of the ensuing cabinet discussions vary but some, such as Young (1989, 300–1), suggest that, while there was vociferous opposition to the proposals, the then Prime Minister, Mrs Thatcher, 'clung on to it [the report] until the majority of ministers told her she had made a terrible mistake'. It may have been a close-run thing but one consequence was the extraction of the government's pledge that the NHS was safe with them, and a diversion of effort into searching for alternative ways of saving money. This did not prevent the government steadily expanding the proportion of NHS funds raised through charges to patients and, in a highly symbolic gesture, ending the practice of free dental and optical checkups, a measure criticised as representing unsound health policy. Even though wholesale privatisation seemed to have been ruled out, the government still appeared to have a

TABLE 8.1 *Typologies of major elements of privatisation in health care in Britain since 1979*

	State	Market	Community
Regulation	Purchaser/provider split. Decentralisation and loss of accountability loosens regulatory grip of health authorities.	Relaxation of consultants' contracts, and of controls on private hospital development. Health authorities encouraged to contract with the private sector, including commercial facilities, for acute care. Localisation of labour regulation.	Social security regulations changed to permit expansion of private nursing homes.
Subsidy	Increased prescription charges. Charging for dental/optical checkups. Tax relief on private health insurance.	Income generation. Land sales to help fund capital programme.	Charitable fundraising to underwrite state provision (eg Great Ormond Street). Charitable contributions to medical research become proportionately more significant.
Provision	Health authorities pulling out of long-stay care. Decline of NHS dentistry. Competitive tendering. Internal markets. Private Finance initiative.	Growth of private health insurance and elective surgery. Rapid expansion of private nursing homes.	Care in the community. More rapid discharge of patients forces more of burden of care onto individuals and families.

number of options, three of which will be discussed here: their encouragement of private health care and of an expansion of charitable funding and provision; the expansion of commercial provision of services within the NHS, including innovations in labour regulation; and the introduction of the internal market mechanisms after the NHS reforms. What we want to show is the way in which privatisation initiatives at first focused on expanding the scope for private provision of services outside the NHS; it then expanded and was at first at the margins of the NHS, being confined to ancillary services; subsequently privatisation moved to the core of the service as attempts were made to mimic market mechanisms throughout the public sector.

Commercial and Charitable Provision of Services

After the 1979 election the Conservatives initially sought to expand the scope for private provision of services outside the NHS. Here their ideological emphasis on freedom of choice attracted support and distanced them from the Labour Party, who when in government had become embroiled in the bitter pay beds disputes of the mid-1970s; the Conservatives could easily characterise Labour's attitude as an interference with freedom. Despite ideological approval of the private sector, the steps taken to encourage its expansion were limited and indirect. Thus there was no tax relief on private health insurance until it was introduced for the elderly in 1991; nor were there attempts to introduce some mechanism for costing and charging for the capital value of NHS assets, which was something persistently demanded by the private sector. Change was confined to minor relaxations of controls on private sector development, and on the time consultants could spend in private practice. Health authorities were encouraged to take account of private provision in developing services and were permitted to contract with commercial hospitals for the first time. In total, though the climate for private sector development was certainly more favourable, representatives of the private sector often felt that the government had not gone as far as they might have done to encourage its expansion (Mohan, 1986). However one crucial change was the innovation in social security regulations, whereby a vast expansion in private sector nursing homes and residential facilities took place, underwritten by the taxpayer. Arguably this signified the first acceptance of the purchaser–provider split in health and social care, and this irretrievably transformed the boundary between the public and private sectors. Finally note that one element in the expansion of private acute care was the greater fragmentation within the labour market, leading to an expansion of private health insurance as companies sought to secure the loyalty of scarce staff with additional fringe benefits.

To some extent such trends could be regarded as separate from government action, since they originated from wider trends in the economy. As for charitable initiatives, these had not disappeared following the establishment of the NHS but their role was marginal, and confined to minor improvements to hospital amenities, although the endowments of the major teaching hospitals remained substantial. At first there was a strategy of limited incrementalism: Patrick Jenkin consistently exhorted health authorities to draw upon the voluntary sector, particularly with respect to community care policy, even though few shared his optimism about the likely extent of community support for hospitals. Health authorities were permitted to engage directly in charitable fund raising and to use Exchequer funds for the purpose. A few hospitals were transferred to the charitable sector, such as the Tadworth Court branch of the Great Ormond Street children's hospital, in 1983, and there were occasional proposals for hospitals to open with a mix of private and NHS funding, thereby broadening the funding base of the hospitals in question, although none of these actually took place. The most significant initiative on these lines was probably the appeal launched in 1988 for the redevelopment of the Great Ormond Street children's hospital; launched with massive media interest and publicity, the appeal easily exceeded its target, but this was in marked contrast to several other appeals which were much less successful (Lattimer and Holly, 1992; Mohan, 1995, ch. 8; Williams, 1989). The success or otherwise of such appeals clearly depended on the 'visibility' of the hospital in question and not on its 'need' or otherwise for funds.

All these initiatives served to redraw the boundary between public and private provision and to create a climate in which private sector expansion and support seemed not only desirable but necessary to secure the future of the NHS. For some Conservative ministers, the travails of the NHS were seen as reflecting the low proportion of health care expenditure funded privately, when compared to other European states; the solution was clearly therefore to enhance the scope for the private sector. Yet the limits to such activities soon became clear: private acute care never reached the coverage of 25 per cent of the population predicted by its more enthusiastic advocates in the early 1980s. Aside from underwriting losses and overcapacity in the hospital sector, expansion was relatively slow, and penetration beyond the professional and managerial socioeconomic groups was limited. Even the introduction of tax relief on insurance premiums for the over-65s, characterised by opponents as the one example of new money in the NHS reforms, did little to change this situation; this was not surprising, given the cost of such premiums, and growth remains sluggish. The private sector has nevertheless made some inroads, especially into elective surgery – up to 25 per cent of such procedures were done privately in the mid-1980s (more recent figures are not available) – but this also reflects the difficulties of the NHS. In the case of long-stay care, finally, the growth in private provision was accompanied by an increase in state regulation as large numbers of new institutions sprang up, but problems of quality and standards remained. The more general point is that this form of privatisation demonstrated that the effect of privatisation measures is not so much to roll back the state as to restructure the character of state intervention, from that of provider to that of purchaser and regulator.

The Entrepreneurial State: the Commercialisation of Health Authority Activity

Despite the expansion of the private sector, it was clear that this would not relieve the NHS of much of its burden, and so health authorities were encouraged to pursue a more entrepreneurial line in seeking resources. In general, the planning guidance issued for the 1982 reorganisation can be seen as marking a shift in tone; Davies (1987) regards this as marking a redefinition of the role of health authorities as an 'entrepreneurial, coordinative' one, pulling together all available sources of care in a locality. The main emphases here included a much more vigorous approach to property management in the NHS, with health authorities being encouraged to identify and dispose of surplus assets and land following the Davies Report (1983). With hindsight this may be regarded as a precursor of the proposals of the 1989 White Paper and also an early response to private sector critics who suggested that competition between NHS and private hospitals was unfair because the private sector had to meet the full cost of its capital whereas in the NHS capital was regarded as a 'free good'. Land sales came to play an increasingly important role in the capital development programme of health authorities, accounting nationwide for up to 24 per cent of the value of the programme in the late 1980s (Health Committee, 1991). However the collapse of the property market in the early 1990s exposed the limitations of this strategy, and left several health authorities coping with major delays in the capital programme.

Health authorities were also encouraged to adopt a more commercial attitude to the exploitation of their assets via the 1987 Health and Medicines Act, which sought to expand income-generating activities. In some respects this built on local initiatives (some health authorities had been operating in the market-place for several years) but what was new was the establishment of an income generation unit within the DoH and the setting of targets for individual health authorities. The whole initiative raised questions of principle and values: was it appropriate that health authorities engaged in such commercial activities, possibly to the detriment of their NHS responsibilities? However, as one prominent general manager pointed out, while the sums involved represented 'peanuts . . . at the moment peanuts are bloody useful' (quoted in Mohan, 1995: 183); in other words the resources available to health authorities left them little alternative.

Clearly not all health authorities had scope to raise income from these various sources, since the potential would depend very much on local conditions and historical accidents (for example, 'assets' in the form of historic buildings, which could be exploited). At some point, given the NHS's labour-intensive nature, market forces would have to be introduced into the determination of labour costs. The first attempt to do this was the introduction of competitive tendering for ancillary services, through which the government intended to signal its determination to challenge union power, open up some elements of wage determination to local labour market forces, expand the scope for private involvement in the health service and restrain costs. The importance of localised determination of wage levels to the government was signalled by the rescission of the Fair Wages Resolution, which had previously required private contractors working in the public sector to comply with public sector terms and conditions of service. The government sought explicitly to prioritise key groups of staff – 'front-line' personnel (medical and nursing staff) over 'support' staff – for example by differential pay awards or through instructions to health authorities to restrain the expansion of the latter group. This was a precursor to a greater degree of marketisation, in the form of proposals for localised pay determination for all staff, which followed the reforms; in this sense market processes had moved from the periphery of the service – influencing remuneration of ancillary staff – to the core, as NHS trusts gained the freedom to determine their own wage levels. Substantial savings were made, though their extent depends on one's definition of costs and benefits. Among the limitations of the scheme, note the following: concerns about service quality, notably with respect to hygiene (Pearson, 1992; Public Services Privatisation Research Unit, 1992; Pollock and Whitty, 1990); limited evidence of competition, as the ancillary service markets came to be dominated by large, often multinational, firms (Mohan, 1991); and problems of labour regulation and labour supply, which contributed to problems of service quality. In respect of labour regulation, some of the limitations of the government's position were exposed in an enquiry into the costs and benefits of privatisation by the Social Services Committee. Union representatives quoted one manager as saying in wage negotiations that he thought the only limitation to competitive tendering was the natural adjustment of market forces; asked how far wages could be reduced, he had replied: 'As far down as you can take it while you still have people coming in to work for you' (Social Services Committee, 1989, Q327). However the corollary was that larger numbers of staff were relying on income support to make up their meagre wages to compensate for the reductions imposed by competitive tendering. Thus money saved by one branch of government was being spent by another.

The Post-reform NHS: Health Providers as 'Flexible Firms'

On a narrow definition, the entities existing in the post-reform NHS might not be said to signify privatisation, for they remained within the public sector. However, in terms of the environment within which they operated, both NHS trusts and fundholding GPs symbolised an important cultural change. Incentive structures had been created in which these bodies were encouraged to pursue public purposes through a *modus operandi* which emphasised private sector values of competition rather than collaboration, with somewhat less regulation than previously.

Thus fundholding GPs, enabled to purchase non-emergency treatment for their patients, have the market power to influence hospital trusts to prioritise their own patients. This, it should be noted, is a quasi-market, for individuals do not make decisions for themselves; rather their doctors intervene to determine where best to send their patients (Bartlett and Le Grand, 1993). Among the consequences have been numerous allegations of priority treatment being given to patients of fundholding practices, and evidence that provider agencies see little alternative but to collaborate in this process if they wish to win the business of fundholders. A related problem is the extent to which fundholders, rather than their patients, capture the benefits of the scheme; on average 60 per cent of savings from fundholding have been used to improve the premises of fundholding doctors, from which GPs themselves may profit personally through selling their practice buildings to other doctors. Even though savings have occurred, it is not clear that fundholding has substantially changed the character of primary health care, nor has it led to significant reductions in waiting times. Thus suspicions remain that simulating market mechanisms in this way leads to familiar problems associated with markets: a failure to respond to social need and the capture of market benefits by producers rather than consumers.

Other problems are evident with NHS trusts. Of course they do have to respond to the demands of purchasers and, given the scale of the NHS budget, this will remain their primary source of income. However numerous trusts have devoted substantial attention to expanding their private business — including the construction of private wings, the better to compete with commercial hospitals — and their income from private sources has grown dramatically since the reforms. Moreover, in acting as autonomous agents in the marketplace, trusts have no incentives to co-operate, so that questions have been raised about the integrated planning of hospital services. If they fail to compete, they can in principle go out of business, as the case of the London hospitals demonstrates (Tomlinson, 1992). This has posed threats to integrated teams of clinicians and researchers, often working across more than one hospital, and depending on each other for the successful prosecution of clinical research. While individual hospitals may in a narrow sense not be 'viable', their activity ought perhaps to be examined in a broader context. Again the fragmentation of the service may be inimical to the pursuit of public ends through the autonomous decisions of individual agencies.

Most recently the announcement of the government's private finance initiative raises the question of the tension between 'planning' and markets which lies at the heart of debates on the NHS (see also Chapter 6 of this volume). Public agencies must now attempt to obtain private sector finance for capital projects and, despite the wealth of historical evidence about underinvestment in health care when it is left to market forces, this also applies to the NHS. The difficulty here is the market disciplines it imposes on trusts, and the consequent effects on their behaviour: will they be tempted to seek the most profitable cases, or to expand the work they do for the private sector, perhaps to the detriment of NHS care? Is it possible that trusts unable to guarantee the volume of patient flow required to underwrite debt servicing will be disadvantaged in bidding for capital funds? If so this would be likely to be against the interests of rural communities and, possibly, of disadvantaged communities likely to offer limited potential for private treatment. Historical parallels are apposite: in the pre-NHS era local authority applications for sanction of loans for capital investment were occasionally rejected by the Ministry of Health on the grounds of the uncertain economic future of the local authorities in question, which would inhibit their ability to repay loans. The effect was to limit the extent to which finance was available in places which arguably needed it most. The private finance initiative arguably brings to an end a long history of co-ordinated, regional planning of hospital development. In future it appears that the trajectory of hospital development will be determined by the autarchic aspirations of individual NHS trusts; gone is a strategic vision for regions as a whole. It is salutary to recall that the proposals for regionalism in the original NHS were born out of frustration with the failures of the previous, essentially market-based, system to provide comprehensive health services distributed more or less equitably.

Market Failures: an Assessment of Privatisation and its Future

This chapter has sought to emphasise the multifaceted nature of privatisation and to stress, what should be obvious, that privatisation measures do not reflect the impress of a single, unitary template, but instead derive from multiple and contradictory motivations. In assessing the impacts of privatisation, it appears undeniable that some initiatives have run up against the limits to recommodification, given the 'market failures' that have emerged. Some of these, more-over, appear inconsistent with the maintenance either of a high-quality service or of a comprehensive one. However, regardless of the scale of privatisation, which in some respects is limited, what may be more important is its effects, in cultural and ideological senses, on the ways in which health care is organised and delivered. This concluding section makes some more general points along these lines.

For some commentators, one effect of the recent changes to the British health care system has been a fragmentation of the NHS into myriad separate entities – trusts, fundholding GPs, private ancillary and consultancy businesses, management buyouts of professional services – each pursuing their own self-interested goals. Greater efficiency in a narrow sense may have resulted, but in a broader sense what appears to have been lost is the relationships of trust and commitment which, for analysts such as Hutton (1995) characterise successful economic organisations. The 'value' released by privatisation measures is often that which is necessary to secure the broader social purposes of the NHS: for instance, greater expenditure on hospital services than that dictated by narrow market conditions may be the price to be paid to ensure the continuance of vital long-term research work; a margin over and above that which is strictly economically necessary may be a price worth paying. Such margins are lost when privatisation proceeds on a purely cost-driven basis. The same may be true for the commercialisation of the NHS: in pursuit of high returns and of income generation, health authorities may dispose of potentially valuable assets, or deploy their existing assets, in ways which would not be the first priority of an equity-seeking service. Reducing every transaction in the NHS to a cost calculus is the most significant internal transformation of the way it operates; it is integral to privatisation; and it is in this sense that a focus on the various antecedents of the NHS reforms is important.

It is important, in addition, to emphasise the limits to privatisation policies as long-term, sustainable solutions to funding crises. The de facto commercialisation of the NHS in fact gives health authorities few options but to reduce labour costs in what is almost a 'palaeo-liberal' conception of the labour market (Jessop, 1991). This is because trusts now must make a guaranteed rate of return on capital assets and, given the high costs of drugs and medical equipment (costs which almost invariably run above the rate of inflation), cutting labour costs is the only significant option available in the health service. Yet this cannot be the basis for a long-term efficiency strategy: standards of quality will inevitably decline and, as the experience of competitive tendering for ancillary services shows, driving costs further and further down eventually brings problems of labour shortages and service interruptions.

Could an alternative be produced? Much of the emphasis in discussions of privatisation has been on commercial providers of services, and these are of course the most visible (and sometimes controversial) players. But some authors have speculated that privatisation might have a progressive potential, leading to a greater degree of community control and participation in service delivery (for example, Donnison, 1985; Lipietz, 1992; Pierson, 1991). There seems little evidence of this in privatisation initiatives in the NHS to date, not least because the internal market offers little to organisations lacking the capitalisation of large commercial operators. Endemic British problems of short-termism (Hutton, 1995) will inhibit the expansion of the British not-for-profit sector, in health care and elsewhere. This is likely to militate against the use of privatisation as a means of restoring democratic control and community accountability in the manner envisaged by Hirst (1993).

A further issue concerns the trade-off between efficiency and equity associated with greater reliance on market forces. If privatisation leads to a position in which greater resources are available in some places than in others, this might contradict the universalist aspirations of the NHS. New Right apologists would see virtue in this, as restoring control to communities and as an escape from the dead hand of bureaucratic regulation, but it may reproduce inequality, albeit on a smaller scale than in the pre-NHS days (and it should not be forgotten that inequalities existed within the NHS anyway). This then leads into wider questions about whether privatisation has produced, or is likely to produce, a *denationalisation* of welfare and a re-emergence of socio-spatial inequalities in service provision. Associated with this are debates about the nature of citizenship: does citizenship entitle one to universal provision of services, or will access to basic services depend on competitive success of individuals or communities in markets? The sociopolitical context of welfare reform proposals is greater social inequality and uneven development within states, combined with questions about the sustainability and affordability of public expenditure commitments at a time of global economic change. The corollary is a greater degree of fragmentation among the electorate, concern about the distributional effects of public expenditure programmes, and the formulation of policies which, explicitly or implicitly, privilege certain key socioeconomic strata. Thus one plausible interpretation of recent health care policy in the UK is in terms of the desire of the Conservative government systematically to prioritise its electoral heartlands in the 'south' over the non-Conservative strongholds of the 'north' (Mohan, 1995: ch. 4). Given the growing evidence of social polarisation in the UK (see Dorling, 1995; Commission on Social Justice, 1994; Rowntree Foundation, 1995) one can anticipate that reform proposals will be framed increasingly with the needs of a 'core' electorate in mind (for a similar argument, see Saltman and von Otter, 1992).

There is a challenge here to arguments which see the welfare state as a genuinely *national* system of institutional arrangements. One of the (implicit) objectives of the welfare state has been the promotion of national social solidarity, but whether such a political project can be sustained seems open to dispute, given the declining ability of the nation state to produce effective central control of economic life while simultaneously the sovereign capabilities of the nation are undermined (Giddens, 1994: 136–40). Equally there may be political limits to the rolling back of state intervention at a time when globalisation is exposing all localities to the chill winds of competition. At issue here is the weakening or elimination of those intermediary institutions which some would regard, even in a market economy, as being essential guarantors of the autonomy of individuals (Gray, 1993). Precisely how (or indeed whether) such tensions are resolved will determine whether the NHS remains one of the more comprehensive and successful public health care systems in the advanced world or whether it becomes merely a safety net for those casualties of the economic insecurity and inequality which currently beset the British economy.

Bibliography

Bartlett, W. and Le Grand, J. (eds) (1993) *Quasi-Markets and Social Policy*, London: Macmillan.

Besley, T. and Gouveia, M. (1994) 'Alternative systems of health care provision', *Economic Policy: A European Forum*, vol. 19, pp. 200–58.

Busfield, J. (1990) 'Social Divisions in Consumption: the case of medical care', *Sociology*, vol. 24, no. 1, pp. 77–96.

Commission on Social Justice (1994) *Social Justice: Strategies for National Renewal*, London.

Davies Report (1983) *Underused and Surplus Property in the NHS*, London: HMSO.

Davies, C. (1987) 'Things to come: the NHS in the next decade', *Sociology of Health and Illness*, vol. 9, pp. 302–17.

Donnison, D. (1984) 'The progressive potential of privatisation', in J. Le Grand and R. Robinson (eds), *Privatisation and the Welfare State*, London: Allen & Unwin.

Dorling, D. (1995) *A New Social Atlas of Britain*, Chichester: Wiley.

Giddens, A. (1994) *Beyond Left and Right: The Future of Radical Politics*, Cambridge: Polity.

Gray, J. (1993) *Beyond the New Right*, London: Routledge.

Green, D. (1994) 'Medical care before the NHS', *Economic Affairs*, vol. 14, no. 5.

Hayek, F. (1944) *The Road to Serfdom*, London: Routledge & Kegan Paul.

Health Committee (1992) *Public Expenditure on Health Matters: Memorandum by the Department of Health*, HC-408, London: HMSO.

Hirst, P. (1993) *Associative Democracy*, Cambridge: Polity.

Hutton, W. (1995) *The State We're In*, London: Cape.

Jessop, B. (1991) 'Thatcherism and flexibility: the white heat of a postfordist revolution', in B. Jessop, H. Kastendiek, C. Neilsen and O. Pedersen (eds), *The Politics of Flexibility*, Aldershot: Edward Elgar.

Jessop, B., Bonnett, K., Bromley, S. and Ling, T. (1987) 'Popular capitalism, flexible accumulation and Left strategy', *New Left Review*, vol. 165, pp. 104–22.

Jessop, B., Bonnett, K., Bromley, S. and Ling, T. (1988) *Thatcherism: A Tale of Two Nations*, Cambridge: Polity.

Johnson, N. (1989) 'The privatisation of welfare', *Social Policy and Administration*, vol. 23, no. 1, pp. 17–30.

Klein, R. and Millar, J. (1995) 'Do-it-yourself social policy', *Social Policy and Administration*, 29(4), 303–16.

Lattimer, M. and Holly, K. (1992) *Charity and NHS reform*, London: Directory of Social Change.

Le Grand, J. and Robinson, R. (eds) (1984) *Privatisation and the Welfare State*, London: Allen & Unwin.

Lipietz, A. (1992) *Towards a New Economic Order: Postfordism, Ecology and Democracy*, Cambridge: Polity.

Marsland, D. (1988) 'The welfare state as a producer monopoly', *Salisbury Review*, vol. 6, pp. 4–9.

Mishra, R (1990) *The Welfare State in Capitalist Society*, Brighton: Harvester Wheatsheaf.

Mohan, J. F. (1986) 'Private medical care and the British Conservative government: what price independence?', *Journal of Social Policy*, vol. 15, pp. 337–60.

Mohan, J. F. (1991) 'The internationalisation and commercialisation of health care in Britain', *Environment and Planning A*, vol. 23, pp. 853–67.

Mohan, J. F. (1995) *A National Health Service? The Restructuring of Health Care in Britain Since 1979*, London: Macmillan.

OECD (1993) *OECD Health Systems: Facts and Trends 1960–1991*, Paris: OECD.

Pearson, M. (1992) 'Health care under Thatcher: pushing the market to its limits?', in P. Cloke (ed.), *Policy and Change in Thatcher's Britain*, Oxford: Pergamon.

Pierson, C. (1991) *Beyond the Welfare State?*, Cambridge: Polity.

Pollock, A. and Whitty, P. (1990) 'Crisis in our hospital kitchens: ancillary staffing during an outbreak of food poisoning in a long-stay hospital', *British Medical Journal*, vol. 300, pp. 383–5.

Powell, M. (1992) 'Hospital provision before the NHS: territorial justice or inverse care law?', *Journal of Social Policy*, vol. 21, pp. 145–63.

Public Services Privatisation Research Unit (1992) *Privatisation: Disaster for Quality*, London: PSPRU.

Redwood, J. (1988) *Popular Capitalism*, London: Routledge.

Rowntree Commission (1995) *Report of the Inquiry into Income and Wealth*, York: Joseph Rowntree Foundation.

Saltman, R. and von Otter, C. (1992) *Planned Markets and Public Competition*, Milton Keynes: Open University Press.

Sharma, U. (1991) *Complementary Medicine Today: Practitioners and Patients*, London: Routledge.

Social Services Committee (1989) Third Report, session 1988–9, Resourcing the NHS: Whitley Councils, IIC-109, London: HMSO.

Tomlinson, B. (1992) *Report of the Inquiry into London's Health Service, Medical Education and Research*, London: HMSO.

Webster, C. (1995) 'Overthrowing the market in health care: the achievements of the early National Health Service', *Journal of the Royal College of Physicians of London*, vol. 29, pp. 502–7.

Williams, I. (1989) *The Alms Trade*, London: Unwin Hyman.

Wistow, G. (1988) 'Offloading responsibilities for care', in R. Maxwell (ed.), *Reshaping the NHS*, Oxford and New Brunswick: Transaction Books.

Young, H. (1989) *One of Us*, London: Macmillan.

9

Conclusion

Nancy North and Yvonne Bradshaw

A range of themes have been introduced and concerns discussed in the preceding chapters, together with differing theoretical explanations of both continuity and change in health care policy. It is worth noting that the issues that have given cause for concern, such as increasing demand for health care, increasing costs of provision and the concomitant search for efficiency savings and cost containment, are not peculiar to health care provision in the UK, but also reflect contemporary concerns with the provision of health care in many other advanced countries. These include the USA, Sweden, the Netherlands, France and Germany, examples from which will be used to illustrate developments later in this chapter.

In this final chapter we pull together some of the material addressed in previous chapters, compare the situation of health care policy in the UK with that of other advanced countries and make some preliminary assessments of the likely way forward for health care policy in the UK. As outlined in Chapters 1 and 3, the establishment of a National Health Service was based on the social democratic principles of universal access to a high-quality, comprehensive system of health care which was collectively funded and provided. These principles appeared to elicit widespread agreement between the two main political parties at this time and the NHS which was formed on the basis of these principles was sustained by a political consensus which continued until the beginning of the 1970s. Despite the subsequent recognition, early in the life of the NHS, that its original aims were not being fully realised, social democrats staunchly defended the principles on which the NHS was based.

However, as discussed in Chapter 1 and subsequent chapters, the criticism of the social democratic-influenced NHS led to both proposed and actual policy changes over time.

One of the most enduring tensions in the development of health care policy in the UK has been that between individualism and collectivism. New Right advocates place particular emphasis on individualism in health care, for both ideological and political reasons, and are strident critics of the type of collectivism which leads to a high level of state provision. The emphasis, from within the New Right, on individual responsibility for health care and the need for cost containment through more efficient use of resources has led them to criticise and subsequently retreat from the universalist/ citizenship model of health care outlined in Chapter 3. Meeting the health care needs of all citizens through universally provided services was a basic principle of the NHS, but, for the New Right, health needs are individualised and personalised and can therefore be better satisfied via the market. Pursuing a minimal model of welfare, involving the privatisation of certain services and the imposition of private sector disciplines in other areas, would, according to the New Right, enable greater freedom for individuals to express their needs and exercise choice as well as concomitantly providing a service which represented value for money (see Chapters 1, 4 and 7).

Unlike those who subscribe to social democratic views, New Right advocates argue that the qualitative difference between health care and consumer goods is not so marked that it necessitates the state's extensive involvement with the provision and, to a lesser degree, the purchase of health care. Some more radical New Right commentators argue that there is no difference at all between health care and other goods normally provided via the market. These beliefs, together with the view that efficiency is inherent in privatisation and the perceived need to contain or even reduce tax-funded expenditure on health care, have led to many changes in health policy, particularly since 1979 when a Conservative government, strongly influenced by the neo-liberal strand of New Right ideology, was elected. However, while free markets in their pure form may have been on the agenda of the radical right, implementation has been constrained by a substantial and entrenched public sector and popular support for the tax-funded NHS. These factors meant that radical shifts towards privatising health care would have been socially and politically untenable. While alternative funding arrangements were considered, for example a change from a taxation-based system to social or private insurance schemes (Butler, 1992), no major changes in the global method of funding the NHS have taken place. What did appear feasible was tackling the organisation of the NHS and creating a quasi-market incorporating managed competition and increasingly pluralistic provision (see Chapters 6 and 8).

Policies of privatisation and advocacy of the minimal state model of health care obviously lay a major stress on individualism and also reflect attempts to contain costs. However if state provision is reduced this will mean that non-state institutions will have to do more. Families, communities, voluntary organisations and the private sector should, according to the New Right, replace state welfare provision where possible. Enhancing the role of the voluntary and informal sectors in the provision of health care and undermining monopolistic state provision are also advocated by welfare pluralists, but in the case of the latter they add the normative proviso that the state should maintain a strategic and regulatory role even though its provider role may be reduced.

It has also been argued, from a number of perspectives, that monopolistic state-provided health care has enabled the medical profession to achieve a degree of power and prestige which allows them to pursue their own self-interest and restrictive practices rather than primarily working for the benefit of society (see Chapters 1 and 5). The problem with the elite position and power of the medical profession is viewed differently from different perspectives. For example, Marxist commentators note their privileged position in the labour market and their involvement with capital accumulation; feminist approaches focus on the gendered division of labour within such professional groups and the treatment of women by the medical profession; those who ascribe to New Right views are more concerned with the way in which the medical profession has maintained its grip on service provision and thus the determination of needs and allocation of resources within the NHS (see Chapter 5). The New Right-influenced policies of the 1980s and 1990s have therefore also been an attempt to undermine the power of the professions in order to implement efficiency savings and thus contain costs. Part of this process has been the extensive use of market rhetoric and the introduction of, albeit modified, market principles. Users of the NHS, who had been cast in the role of passive consumers of services, which were determined and allocated by the medical profession, were to be given greater freedom of choice within the developing quasi-market for health care.

However it was not only the New Right who were critical of the way in which the NHS operated. From the 1970s, the paternalism and bureaucratic insensitivity which appeared to be inherent features of the NHS were challenged from a number of directions. The political left were critical of the lack of responsiveness to service users within the NHS and called for greater decentralisation, democratic participation and accountability as a solution to the disempowerment of service users, rather than attempting to enhance consumer sovereignty through further forms of privatisation. However, whether the preferred solution to the problems of the NHS is to increase the relative power of the consumer or to promote greater democratic participation, neither path is problem-free, as Chapter 7 clearly identifies.

With the publication of *Working for Patients* in 1989, Margaret Thatcher made it quite clear that the preferred aim of the government was to promote consumerism rather than democracy as the means of achieving a more patient-responsive cost-efficient health care service. Democracy had not been removed from the New Right agenda, but this was to take the form of enfranchisement of individuals via the market rather than the more traditional form of participatory democracy advocated by those on the political left. Despite the rhetoric of consumer responsiveness the consumerism pursued was to be a collectivised form limiting individual consumers to the exercise of choice in the selection of GPs, or to the expression of their opinions via a complaints mechanism. It would seem that individual consumers have gained little from the implementation of quasi-markets, wherein it is the purchasers of health care who act as proxy consumers. The levels of democratic participation and accountability within the NHS have arguably never been high, even at its inauguration in 1948, but the remodelling of health authorities along the lines of private sector boards of directors, in the process removing local authority representatives and Community Health Councils' speaking rights, appears to have further reduced the semblance of democracy that existed previously.

A change which is perhaps of greater significance is that brought about in attitudes and values, not only by the marketisation of the NHS, but also by the market rhetoric and ideology of privatisation which has been a concomitant of the reforms since 1979. As John

Mohan points out in Chapter 8 of this volume, the cultural and ideological dimensions of privatisation may lead to the legitimisation of competitive behaviour which is aimed at gaining private benefits and create the conditions in which people prioritise individualist solutions and thus seek to exit from the collectively provided NHS. These types of changes again reflect the continuing tension between individual and collective interests.

The motivations for pursuing policies of privatisation and the constraints on this process which have resulted in quasi-markets may have their roots in economic growth and the evolution of more discerning, self-reliant citizen-consumers. It could be argued, however, that to fully understand the form that privatisation has taken in the UK necessitates an examination of the political sphere. Elsewhere health care systems have established more pluralistic arrangements for the financing, administration and provision of health care and can accordingly be described as more privatised. This does not mean that they have escaped the difficulties facing the UK and, indeed, in some instances, broadly similar remedies have been applied. In contrast, some states have sought to ameliorate the negative effects of a marketised health care system, attempting to introduce measures which broaden access to health care.

The type of policies adopted by a country in response to concerns about or crises within health care provision will reflect the particular historical development of health care provision, the culture of institutions involved, the dominant political ideology and the current economic situation. Given the caution which should accompany diverse accounts of health care systems – it must be borne in mind that policies cannot simply be transferred from one country to another and be expected to work in the same way – it is nevertheless a useful exercise to examine their responses in relation to the themes explored in this and other chapters.

The problem of medical price inflation, the rising expectations of an increasingly sophisticated health care 'consumer' and increasing proportions of elderly people in western Europe and North America have meant that existing standards of health care provision have been placed under pressure as governments have attempted to control the amount of public and private spending on health care. Inevitably this is easier to achieve in the former. According to de Roo (1995), as social health care schemes fail to keep up with what is technically available, additional inequalities between private and public schemes will evolve.

Whatever the purported advantages of a marketised health care system (productive efficiency, allocative efficiency and greater consumer satisfaction), the ensuing inequalities ultimately challenge social solidarity. In the Netherlands a fairly complex system of health care funding operates in which individuals below a certain threshold income are compulsorily insured for acute care in schemes administered by sickness funds. Contributions are income-dependent, but the schemes are also partly funded from tax revenues. The remaining 40 per cent of the population may take out private insurance for acute care requirements or pay providers directly. Other categories of care, such as child health care, mental health care and long-term care needs, are funded from universal compulsory health insurance, subsidised by taxation. Dissatisfaction with these arrangements arose, in part, because of the perceived unfairness whereby actuarily sensitive private insurance schemes offer lower premiums to certain categories of insurees while their less well off counterparts are obliged to pay higher premiums within the compulsory insurance schemes. In the context of these and other difficulties the Dekker Committee was asked by the Netherlands' government to examine the health care system. Amongst other measures, it proposed a compulsory insurance system for all the population, based on income-related contributions. These would be pooled in a central fund which would distribute risk-associated premiums to the insuring agency selected by the individual consumer. The remainder of the premium would be paid by the insuree; each insurer would charge the same rate to all individuals subscribing to that particular agency, although insurers would compete over the price and content (for example, the contracted providers) of the insurance package offered. Voluntary supplementary insurance would also be available.

The Dekker proposals, which were later amended slightly in the 1990 Simons Plan, thus sought to develop a unified system of basic health insurance (OECD, 1992), thereby adopting a more collectivist solution to the problems of financing health care, although de Roo argues that the income-related premiums still impose disproportionate costs on lower-income groups. This argument has yet to be tested, for other elements in the proposals generated opposition from pressure groups, namely from the sickness funds, the medical profession and the hospital sector. The current government policy is for a scaled down coverage of the mandatory insurance scheme, nevertheless covering the essential elements of ambulatory, hospital and long-term care, which will be introduced incrementally.

Political opposition in the USA also resulted in the collapse of other proposals which would have ushered in a more collectivist approach to health care. The USA's health system is largely funded from private sector payments (corporate schemes and individual insurance) although the public sector contribution to health care funding has increased dramatically since Medicare and Medicaid were introduced in 1965, notwithstanding the subsequent attempts of administrations to constrain costs. In particular, regulations governing access to the Medicaid programme, which funds care for low-income families with children and certain categories of disabled, the cost of which is shared by both Federal and state governments, have become increasingly restrictive. The absence of compulsory health care insurance leaves some 30 million of the population medically indigent, according to Ham *et al.* (1990). As well as the unemployed, the uninsured population includes low income workers and their families.

The Clinton health care reforms proposed to reduce the less desirable outcomes of a market in health care. These were the unwanted transaction costs (for example, administration and advertising costs), the relatively limited access described above and the problems of adverse selection (where insurers or providers avoid high-risk and potentially costly individuals). The Clinton proposals involved establishing regional health alliances which in addition to large companies, would be able to purchase health care for their population or, in the case of companies, their workforce. Individuals insured by the health alliances would be responsible for 20 per cent of the cost of a weighted average premium, with the poor being fully subsidised and therefore able to enjoy a level of health care similar to that of a large proportion of the population (Wiener, 1995). Clinton's proposals for health care reform, and thus for a more collectivist approach to health care, albeit within a steadfastly pluralistic system of provision, failed to gain the support of key pressure groups, including the American Medical Association, and ultimately of Congress. Some of the objections raised related to the perceived costs of administering a scheme to subsidise large numbers of individuals, the resulting possibility of tax increases and the increased involvement of government. As Wiener suggests, 'Americans have low regard for their governments and do not want to see them play a more important role' (1995: 129), evidence of the significance of political culture for policy processes.

Both the above initiatives were attempts to address imperfections in previous arrangements for health care which attempted to collectivise coverage. In the case of the USA, the Clinton proposals were a radical initiative, given previous approaches to the welfare state. However both the Clinton and the Dekker proposals attempted to address other inefficiencies in the systems. The Dekker/Simons plan in the Netherlands also sought to create more flexibility in the system and more choice for consumers. Its solution was to discourage the territorial monopolies created by the benefit funds and promote competition between insurers in both the voluntary and commercial sectors. Although insurers would receive risk-adjusted per capita payments from a central fund and would compete over the price and content of insurance packages, the same rate would be charged to each insuree choosing that contract. Sickness funds are not allowed to reject applicants, thus 'cream skimming' of the youngest and fittest patients was to be avoided. The increased competition amongst insurers, it was argued, would lead to greater discretion when contracting with providers and thus improved productive efficiency and quality of care. Although the reforms are being introduced slowly and it is too early to evaluate them comprehensively, initial indications are that providers are adjusting their activities and concentrating on improving the quality of their performance (Van de Ven and Schut, 1995).

Sweden provides an example of a state where parallels with the UK are more tangible. The Swedish welfare state, founded on principles of universality and social solidarity, developed to the point where it consistently had one of the highest levels of public expenditure amongst OECD states (Olsson and McMurphy, 1993). Criticism of an unresponsive and bureaucratic welfare state in the late 1960s, coupled with the destabilising effects of economic recession, created a lack of confidence in welfare policies. The return of a conservative coalition government in the mid-1970s saw the beginning of a reform process in which decentralisation, privatisation and a restructuring of welfare provision were high on the political agenda. Against this broad, revisionist backcloth, more specific criticisms of the health service identified inefficiencies in provision, including an overdependence on hospital based care, a lack of choice for consumers and public providers who were insulated by their near-monopoly position and thus uninspired to change things.

In Sweden responsibility for financing and managing health care services lies with 26 county councils, who also own most health care facilities. The reforms, over which county councils have exercised individual discretion, have mainly attempted to strengthen consumer choice. By 1993 all county councils offered free choice of primary health centre and most offered a choice of hospital. This has encouraged the further development of private health care centres. In most places payments followed patients (Anell, 1996), thus creating incentives for providers to compete for patients. Anell reports that the threat of contestability was sufficient to induce changes in providers, just as has occurred in the Netherlands. Furthermore, by 1993 eight county councils had separated purchaser–provider functions; in some models the purchasing function had been devolved to primary care level, an obvious similarity to GP fundholding in the UK. Anell suggests, however, that overall the degree of purchaser–provider separation is weak compared with that in the UK.

Thus it is evident from these examples that market remedies, creating or enhancing competition, have been the favoured solution for several European states, although the UK has had to create, as far as possible, a plurality of separate providers and purchasers from previous monolithic administrative systems. The quest for productive efficiency has been one very obvious objective in all the reform processes discussed so far, but in addition there have been nationally focused concerns related to access (the Clinton proposals) and equitable distribution of costs (the Netherlands). In the case of the UK, Sweden and the Netherlands, universal access to adequate health care was an accepted principle of the various systems, which nevertheless had all been criticised for their monolithic and inflexible forms of provision.

The improvement of consumer choice is, of course, a rationale for markets, though arguably both Sweden and the Netherlands have placed a higher priority on this than the UK government (see Chapter 7). Quite clearly, however, markets reduce or eliminate choice for those whose care is insufficiently subsidised. In France regulations which permitted doctors the option of setting their own fees over and above the fee schedule (a part of which is reimbursed to patients) had by 1990 resulted in the majority of doctors in the major cities operating on this basis. Less well-off patients found it difficult to find public sector doctors whose charges remained within the nationally agreed schedule.

However choice through diversity is not the only consumerist approach. Improving the quality of information, creating standards which help to establish a framework of patient rights, clarifying insurer and/or provider responsibilities and simplifying complaints procedures are all important factors reinforcing the relatively weak position of service users. This is no simple endeavour: 'No one doubts that competing providers will have the incentive to present an *image* of high quality care, but it is the *reality* that will matter' (OECD; 1992: 99, original emphasis). Countries such as the Netherlands have well-developed mechanisms for quality assurance established by both government and insurers. The expectation is that agencies monitoring provider quality, such as certification institutes, will extend this further, (OECD, 1992). In contrast, Anell (1996) suggests that information which would allow Swedish health care users to make comparisons between providers has not generally been available; some studies have revealed that consumers are not even aware of the choices on offer.

The health care systems of European countries such as France, Germany, Belgium and the Netherlands are more pluralistic than those of the UK and Sweden, but this fact has not necessarily resulted in cost-effectiveness. In addition to what might be described as a macroeconomic remedy, the encouragement of greater competition, most governments have intervened to control health care costs. The measures available to governments vary. Where they have direct involvement in provision, as in France and Sweden, it is possible to impose fixed, prospective budgets on hospital services. France has operated this system for all hospitals involved in public health care provision (that is, all public hospitals and some voluntary institutions) since 1985. During the 1980s the county councils in Sweden devolved health care management to district level, each with a global budget. One reason for the low costs (expressed as a proportion of GDP) of the NHS has been the capacity of central government to set global budgets for regional health authorities. Since the 1990 reforms these have gradually been reallocated at the level of district health authorities. In the USA third party insurers have refined prospective budgeting further with the use of Diagnostic Related Groups whereby hospitals are paid a fixed price according to the patient's diagnosis.

Other measures in the armoury of purchasers are intended to be more precise in their effect. Patient co-payments extracted at the time of treatment are not only intended as a source of revenue, but also attempt to discourage cavalier consumption. In France patients pay a fixed proportion of the fee for ambulatory care (GP or hospital outpatient) and for any prescribed medication. Hospital care is also charged, but the cost is mainly paid by the *caisses* or sickness funds. In Germany the co-payments for inpatient care rose by 50 per cent in 1991 and patient transport charges have also increased. Privatising the cost of health care is also evident in the increases in the proportion of compulsory health contributions deducted from income occurring in Belgium, Germany and France. Similarly in the USA increased premiums and co-payments for Medicare represent a rise in the proportion of costs underwritten by patients.

The drive to control costs in the USA and Europe has resulted in governments and third party insurers introducing measures which directly affect the medical profession. In France and Sweden restraints on salaries of doctors within the public sector have meant that both governments have had to permit doctors to cultivate private practice, but with different results. As noted before, in France this effectively has severely limited choices for some patients in cities. By contrast the out of hours private enterprise of some Swedish doctors, which is still funded by the state, has created additional primary care provision and competition for public providers. In the USA corporate health maintenance organisations employ salaried physicians (who thus have no incentive to overtreat as with fee-for-service payments) and may provide monetary incentives to remain within budgets.

Other measures involve more of a direct challenge to the autonomy of the medical profession. As in the UK, there has been increasing interest in ensuring that doctors practise cost-effective medicine. Without question, health care in the USA has led the way in the surveillance of medical practice. Utilisation reviews of patient treatment plans are designed to weed out unnecessary investigations and treatments or any which might fall outside treatment protocols. In France, where the tradition of *médicine libérale* (a concept protective of clinical autonomy and the primacy of the doctor–client relationship) has produced a strong medical profession, the government has required doctors' representatives and the sickness funds to negotiate fee schedules for treatments which in turn are expected to demonstrate cost-effectiveness. In Germany quality assurance programmes are being introduced following discussions between sickness funds and medical associations. Detailed arrangements were to be left to the parties concerned but it is likely that this would involve some form of utilisation review.

The prescribing of pharmaceutical products has become a popular target amongst European states where effort has been focused on restricting the range of products available on state-subsidised prescriptions. Generic prescribing (of the chemical rather than the trade name of a product) enables pharmacists to dispense less expensive products; this is encouraged in both the UK and Germany. In France, as in the UK, the prescribing habits of GPs are monitored and pressure is brought to bear on those with excessive practices. France and the UK also restrict the availability of drugs available on 'public' prescription to those deemed effective.

These and other measures which in some way attempt to control the way doctors work have not been introduced without opposition. They are precisely aimed methods of altering professional behaviour and have been represented by the profession as unnecessary and damaging incursions on the doctor–patient relationship. No doubt the resentment is also due to the fact that these mechanisms are dissolving the autonomous position of the medical profession. However they should not be seen in isolation from macro-level processes, chief amongst which is the injection of more competitive environments. Speaking of the UK medical profession Berwick *et al.* suggest that 'no door bolts tightly enough to exclude the realities that have come to besiege modern medicine' (1992: 235), a quote equally relevant to medical brethren elsewhere. Nevertheless the profession retains a powerful position in policy bargaining processes in European states and has proved capable of attenuating the effects or slowing the implementation of policy. As essential participants in the delivery of health care they will continue to play a major role in policy development.

The chapter so far has shown that concerns about the increasing demand for health care have motivated a number of European states to embark on health care policies which variously attempt to control costs, enhance provider efficiency and enable consumer choice. Differences in prioritisation of these objectives and, more importantly, the strategies they adopt are a product of a country's political culture and its historic approach to welfare provision. Thus, while it is possible to detect similar broad principles, such as the encouragement of actual or threatened competition between providers, the manifestation of these in national health policies varies just as the measures themselves are applied to distinctive health care systems.

What is also apparent is that fairly radical changes conceptualised by policy makers emerge in a more evolutionary fashion. The Dekker/ Simons blueprint in the Netherlands is being introduced in a piecemeal manner because of the difficulties of marshalling the support of key interest groups such as the municipal assurance companies and the medical profession (Elsinga, 1989). Similarly Anell (1996) describes inconsistencies in the Swedish reforms, with local politicians reluctant to deviate too much from an integrated model of health care provision and a lack of real rewards for providers who attract additional patients.

By these standards the NHS reforms over the last decade and a half have been comprehensive in their execution and potentially radical in outcome. Various authors in this book have already commented on the changed culture of the NHS, the blurring of private and public sector provision, the reforms' impact on professional groups and the increasing emphasis on individual responsibility for health. Whether or not these broad trends continue and strengthen in the medium term may depend on the policies of the next government, to be elected in 1997.

If the Conservatives regain office it is likely that present policies, which seek to encourage a contestable market in health care, will continue, although indications are that there is likely to be an attempt to consolidate rather than promote new policies. The extension of GP fundholding to allow multi-funds to develop total purchasing for the practices' populations and the hitherto hesitant practices to experience a limited form of fundholding, covering prescribing costs and the purchase of community nursing services (NHSE, 1994), will further entrench this, the most radical aspect of the 1990 reforms. This will further erode the purchasing function of the new health authorities, created in April 1996 from district health authorities and the family health service authorities, although they will continue to retain certain purchasing responsibilities for at least a majority of the population.

Notwithstanding the successes of fundholding noted by the Audit Commission (1996a) which included reducing waiting list times and more responsiveness from hospital services, the same assessment raised questions about the overall cost-effectiveness of fundholding. In

1994/5, the average fundholder made savings of £53 000 with 24 per cent of underspending fundholders saving £100 000 or more (Audit Commission, 1996b). Year on year savings of this nature, which are invested in practice capital and services, raise concerns about inequality of local provision. Practice-based staffing, information technology and other equipment costs were assessed as £232m. Health authorities' administrative costs were put at an additional £6000 per annum per fundholding practice, along with the extra administrative burden placed on trusts who have to negotiate contracts with a multiplicity of purchasers (Audit Commission, 1996a). A government pledged to reduce unnecessary administrative overheads cannot afford to overlook these figures, especially since on this basis further expansion of the number of fundholders would increase, perhaps to intolerable levels, the pressure on health authority budgets.

In their policy brief for health care, *Renewing the NHS*, the Labour Party have criticised the transaction costs of the internal market, including the costs of administering fundholding. Stating that 'GP fundholding as it currently stands is unacceptable' (1995: 30), they propose area or locality commissioning, involving all GPs in health care planning. One suggestion which appears to flirt with fundholding is the use of pilot 'shadow budgets': money allocated on a weighted capitation basis is managed by the health authority on behalf of one or more practices, who may then negotiate with local providers to improve services. The aim is to encourage cost transparency and innovation with administrative economies of scale and strategic control.

The dilution rather than the negation of current Conservative health policies is evident in other proposals. The separation of functions, with health authorities continuing in a planning and development role and hospitals and other services focusing on service delivery, would continue, but the more aggressive aspects of the internal market would be tempered. Yearly contracts, for example, would be replaced by Comprehensive Healthcare Agreements (CHAs) with local health services (LHS). The CHAs would also enable patients from other health authorities to use services, reverting to the pre-internal market system. The regional administrative tier would be responsible for modifying funding allocations to districts based on cross-boundary flows. The authorities themselves would be constituted from 'specialists' in health and social care as well as 'generalists'. This terminology could signal the reinstatement of hospital clinicians on critical decision-making bodies, although a stronger GP presence is more likely. Thus the medical profession in its entirety will be rehabilitated within policy processes, although these will be more pluralistic, representing a balance between the primary and secondary care sectors. In the Labour Party model, health authorities would assume a more central role in the planning of services, a logical extrapolation of health authorities' role alongside fundholding being a source of intelligence on health needs and cost-efficiency and a loose orchestrator of fundholder purchasing to satisfy strategic needs.

In a NHS under a Labour government co-operation would replace competition, but the performance of the medical profession within the LHS will continue to come under increasing scrutiny. In an attempt to improve cost-efficiency, comparative assessments of costs between hospitals will be introduced; future possibilities include resource allocation using human resource groups, the ascribing of treatment costs according to pre-designated cost bands. Clinical audit has a place in both Conservative and Labour Parties' plans for the NHS, with the latter promoting practice audits for primary care. This increase in surveillance of clinical practice will further limit professional autonomy, a process identified in Chapter 5).

Labour envisages a far more active role for patients and their representatives, with strengthened community health councils monitoring provision in hospital and community services and GP practices and a return to the concept of local authority participation in health care agreements. As well as having a changed terminology the boards of trusts would be replaced by new governing bodies of the LHS constituted from patients' groups, members of professional and staff organisations and the voluntary sector, a more pluralistic local policy-making process. Other than this, recommendations are remarkably similar to the intentions of the present Conservative government: a concern to simplify the complaints procedure and create clear standards of care, which strengthen the rights of the *individual* patient within the system.

The role of private financing and private medicine is not rejected in Labour's agenda for the NHS, but predictably is dealt with cautiously. The most unequivocal statement relates to compulsory competitive tendering, which is to be ended. While not confirming a total reversal of the Conservative government's private capital initiative, discussed in Chapter 8, the Labour Party signals its displeasure and proclaims its intention to disallow private sector 'cherry picking' of particular contracts (1995: 26). Similarly private medicine using NHS premises and resources is to be examined to ensure the public sector is adequately recompensed and waiting times for treatments are not adversely affected. The Conservatives, however, are likely to encourage private investment in trusts' capital developments and the further blurring of public and private provision of services.

This prospectus for the NHS does not therefore signify massive change. In the scale of events of the last 17 years, since the Conservatives gained power in 1979, what might be undertaken by either a Labour or Conservative government will propel the NHS along a similar trajectory. There will continue to be a defined separation of functions between health authorities and current providers, with the former controlling resources. The present emphasis on efficiency, particularly in respect of evidence based clinical practice, and on a strategic planning process which involves GPs and possibly other stakeholders will continue. The patient as consumer will continue to exercise little choice but may find that others will represent his or her interests more effectively than in the past.

The pursuit of better value for money health care linked to the ever-expanding areas of medical intervention will of necessity lead to the setting of priorities. Whether this prioritisation takes place at a national level, or is devolved to local agencies operating within national guidelines, will significantly affect consumer choice in terms of treatment, as well as determining who will exercise power and influence in decision making.

Within both the health care system of the UK and those of other countries, it would seem that the broad trends and patterns, outlined in this and preceding chapters, are unlikely to be reversed. While this chapter can only speculate on the future of health care provision, there is likely to be encouragement of a mixed economy in health care, a greater emphasis placed on the role of primary care, and cost efficiency and effectiveness will continue to occupy a primary place on the political agenda; linked to these will be continuing incursion on the autonomy of the medical profession. As this final chapter has shown, countries will identify different sets of priorities and embark on strategies which to some extent reflect their political heritage, the constraints of current welfare organisation, and which are ultimately determined by the politics of implementation.

Bibliography

Anell, A. (1996) 'The monopolistic integrated model and health care reform: the Swedish experience', *Health Policy*, vol. 37, pp. 19–33.

Audit Commission (1996a) *What the Doctor Ordered*, London: HMSO.

Audit Commission (1996b) *Fundholding Facts*, London: HMSO.

Berwick, D. M., Enthoven, A. and Bunker, J. P. (1992) 'Quality Management in the NHS: the doctor's role–1, *British Medical Journal*, vol. 304, pp. 235–9.

Butler, J. (1992) 'Patients, Policies and Politics', *Before and after Working for Patients*, Buckingham: Open University Press.

de Roo, A. A. (1995) 'Contracting and Solidarity: Market-Oriented Changes in Dutch Health Insurance Schemes', in *Implementing Planned Markets in Health Care*, Buckingham: Open University Press.

Elsinga, E. (1989) 'Political decision-making in health care: the Dutch case', *Health Policy*, vol. 11, pp. 243–55.

Ham, C., Robinson, R. and Benzeval, M. (1990) *Health Check: Healthcare Reforms in an International Context*, London: King's Fund Institute.

Klein, R. (1995) *The New Politics of the NHS*, London: Longman.

Labour Party (1995) *Renewing the NHSL Labour's Agenda for a healthier Britain*, London: Labour Party.

NHSE (1994) *Developing NHS Purchasing and GP Fundholding* (EL (94) 79), Leeds: NHS Executive.

OECD (1992) *The Reform of Health Care. A comparative analysis of seven OECD countries*, Paris: OECD.

Olsson, S. V. and McMurphy, S. (1993) 'Social policy in Sweden: the Swedish model in transition', in R. Page and J. Baldcock (eds), *Social Policy Review 5*, Canterbury: Social Policy Association.

Van de Ven, W. P. M. M. and Schut, F. T. (1995) 'The Dutch experience with internal markets', in M. Jerome-Forget, J. White and J. M. Wiener (eds), *Health Care Reform Through Internal Markets*, Montreal: Institute for Research on Public Policy; Washington: The Brookings Institution.

Wiener. J. M. (1995) 'Managed competition as financing reform: a view from the United States', in M. Jerome-Forget, J. White and J. M. Wiener (eds), *Health Care Reform Through Internal Markets*, Montreal: Institute for Research on Public Policy; Washington: The Brookings Institution.

Index

accumulation   see capital accumulation
Acheson Report   121
acute care, private   159, 160
AHAs   see Area Health Authorities
Alford's study of health care   35–8
   applied to NHS   38
Alma Ata declaration   133–4
alternative therapies   92
anti-racist perspectives   17–20
approved societies   53
Area Health Authorities (AHAs)   63
   abolition of   97
Asian workers   18
audit
   and litigation   145
   medical   103
autonomy, clinical   24–5

Belgium   179, 180
Bevan, Aneurin   57–8, 95
Beveridge Report   3–4, 56
black people
   discrimination in medical school and
      hospital post-admissions   134–5
   status in labour force   18
Black Report   72, 73
BMA   see British Medical Association
BPM (Bureaucratic/Organisational
   Process Model)   31
Bradbeer Report   96–7
British Medical Association (BMA)
   and National Health Insurance   52
   and NHS formation   56–7, 59, 94
Brown plan   56–7
bureaucracies
   in NHS   99–100, 104, 105
   welfare   130, 131
Bureaucratic/Organisational Process
   Model (BPM)   31

capital, social   14, 15
capital accumulation
   function of state   14, 15
   role of medicine in   88, 89

capitalism
   Marxist views   13–15, 33–4
   and racism   18
centralisation
   encouraged by reforms   126
   see also decentralisation
Central Policy Review Staff
   (CPRS)   156
Centre for NHS Reviews and
   Dissemination   122
charitable provision of services   158–60
CHAs (Comprehensive Healthcare
   Agreements)   183
CHCs (Community Health
   Councils)   64, 135–6, 137, 140–1
childbirth, feminist perspectives   12
choice, individuals' freedom of   70
Citizen's Charter   92
citizenship
   and collectivism   74
   conferring entitlement to
      services?   166
   welfare rights   74, 75
Clinton proposals (USA)   176–7, 178
Cochrane Centres   122
collectivism   67, 71–4
   and citizenship   74
   v. individualism   171
   post-war political expediency   72
   social organisations   72
   and welfare pluralism   67, 74
collegiate professional power   87
commercial provision of
   services   158–60
communities, welfare role of   77, 78
community, as group in health care
   study   35, 37
community-based services   62
Community Health Councils
   (CHCs)   64, 135–6, 137, 140–1
complaints   145
complementary therapies   92
Comprehensive Healthcare Agreements
   (CHAs)   183

comprehensiveness 4, 9
consensus management, 1974 health
    service reorganisation 97
Conservatism
    modern values 7
    neo-conservatism 7, 113
consultants, conditions of service 103–4
consultation with public 142–4
consumer choice 117–18, 120, 126–7
consumerism
.   danger of popularist prioritising 143
    information and consultation 141–4
    principles 132–3, 141–2
    user criticism affected by client
        vulnerability 144
consumerism and democracy 131–4
    before 1979 134–6
    after 1979 136–41, 173
consumer law 131–2
consumers
    assertiveness 92
    increasing expectations 174
    proxies 139
    see also consumer choice
corporate rationalisers 35, 36
cost analyses 120–1
costs
    curbs on management costs 105
    escalation 8, 60–1, 69–70, 78
    medical price inflation 174
    savings 162, 165–6
cost shifting 69–70, 126, 154–5, 156
CPRS (Central Policy Review
    Staff) 156

Davies Report 160
decentralisation, administrative 133,
    138
decision making
    Bureaucratic (Organisational) Process
        model (BPM) 31
    control methods 26–7
    co-opting potential opposition 27
    exclusion of minority interests 26
    flawed theories 29
    rationality in 28–9
    routines in 31
    see also policy making
Dekker Committee (Netherlands) 175,
    177, 182
democracy
    and the NHS 136
    see also consumerism and democracy

dental checkups 156
DHAs *see* District Health Authorities
Diagnostic Related Groups (USA) 179
District Health Authorities
        (DHAs) 139
    policy interpretation 24
'diswelfare' 5
doctors
    conflicts among 35–6, 93
    hegemony challenged 92, 102
    importance of individualism 68
    influence over health policy 94–7
    junior 93
    loss of power? 88
    NHS concessions to 95
    role in NHS 86
    see also general practitioners;
        professionals

economic growth
    and privatisation 152
    and welfare policies 5–6
economic liberalism 6
efficiency, and market discipline 126
elderly people, status of services
    for 61–2
elite theory 35
Emergency Medical Services (Second
    World War) 55
employer-based welfare schemes 76
empowerment
    of consumers 131–4
    individual *v.* collective 74
    see also power
entrepreneurialism 160–2
epidemiological training and
    assessment 121–2, 123, 125
ethnic minorities
    consultation with 142
    disadvantaged position 17, 18, 20
    immigration control 18, 19
    a problem? 18–19
    as scapegoats? 18
    special needs of 19
    stereotypical views of 19–20
    as welfare producers 20
evidence-based medicine 122
Evidence-Based Medicine (journal) 122
exclusionary closure 88–9, 89–90
expenses, social 14, 15

Fair Wages Resolution 161
families, welfare role of 77–8

Family Health Service Authorities   139
Family Practitioner Committees
   (FPCs)   137
feminism and feminist perspectives   1–2,
   9–12, 34
   ambivalence   9–10
   on childbirth   12
   critique of the professions   89–91
   gender concept   1
   liberal feminism   10, 34
   linked with collectivism   67
   Marxist-feminism   34–5
   on medical model of health care   12
   radical feminism   11, 34
   socialist feminism   10–11
finance alternatives   113, 115, 156
First Green Paper   62–3, 64
FPCs (Family Practitioner
   Committees)   137
France   178–9, 180, 181
free market   111–13
   problems   3
Friendly Societies   49, 53, 77
   health care   51
fundholding   *see* general practitioner
   fundholding
funding alternatives   113, 115, 156

general management   70–1, 98–9
general practitioner fundholding   125,
   126, 140, 143, 162–3
   benefits gained by?   163
   cost-effectiveness   182–3
   successes   182
general practitioners
   capitation fees   138
   choice of and changing   134–5, 138–9
   contracts   103
   deregistering patients   139
   provider power   139
   as purchasers   139
   see also doctors; general practitioner
      fundholding; professionals
Germany   180, 180–1, 181
GPs   *see* general practitioners
Great Ormond Street children's
   hospital   159
Griffiths Report   43, 70–1, 98–100, 137
   attempt to limit medical
      power   98–100
   impact on nursing profession   99
   introduction of general
      management   98–100

medical response to   99
occupational culture and
   management   99–100
philosophy of   98

halo effect   144
health, individual responsibility for
   own   133–4
Health and Medicines Act 1987   161
health authorities
   administrative costs   183
   charitable fund raising   159
   as entrepreneurs   160–2
   land sales   160–1
   tasks   139–40
health care
   different from consumer goods?   5,
      75–6
   effect of industrialisation   49–50
   influences on supply of   132
   inter-war years   53–4
   minimal state model   48, 67, 78
   nineteenth century   48–50, 75
   non-state   48–9
   pluriform system   127
   pre-NHS overlapping and
      inefficiencies in   55
   price barrier to?   6
   rationing of   123, 124
   Second World War   55
   social insurance model   51, 56
   state *v.* non-state roles   52, 67
   universalist/citizenship model   53–6,
      59–62, 65, 67, 78
   women as users and providers of   10,
      12
   see also hospitals; National Health
      Service; voluntary sector; *and*
      individual countries
health care planning, Alford's
   study   35–8
Health Education Council   71
health insurance
   insurance companies, and NHI   53
   insurance schemes, NHS   115
   obstacles to systems of   156
   see also National Health Insurance;
      private health insurance; *and*
      individual countries
health maintenance organisations
   (HMOs)   115
Health of the Nation   70, 122
Healthy Cities approach (WHO)   74

HMOs (health maintenance
    organisations) 115
home help services 54
Hospital Plan (1962) 59–60
hospitals
    charitable funds for 159
    local government 50, 54
    Poor Law infirmaries 51
    teaching hospitals 58–9
    voluntary 49, 50, 54–5, 57, 77

iatrogenesis, levels of 91
immigration control 18, 19
incrementalism 29–30, 40, 159
independence, through privatisation 154
indigent 132
individualism 67, 68–71
    v. collectivism 171
    collectivist critique of 73
    importance to clinicians 68
    and the New Right perspective 67,
        68–9
indoor relief 48, 49
industrialisation 49–50
    effect on professionals 85
information giving 141–2
institutional model of state welfare *see*
    universalist/citizenship model
insurance *see* health insurance
internal market 116–17, 138
    see also providers; purchasers
issue networks 39, 40, 140

labour cost reduction 165–6
Labour Party, health care policy 183–5
labour regulation 162
land sales 160–1
learning difficulties, status of
    services 61–2
legitimation function of state 14
LHS (local health services) 183, 184
liberal feminism 10, 34
life-style choices 68–9, 70
litigation 145
Local Government Act 1929 54
local government hospitals 50, 54
local health services (LHS) 183, 184
Local Voices 140, 141–2, 143

management
    cost curbs 105
    general 70–1, 98–9
    scientific approaches 101

managers, professional, in NHS
    accountable to Government 101, 106
    Griffiths report 98–100
    rise of 100–1
    traits 101
marketising the NHS 114–18
markets
    egalitarian and democratic? 153
    regulation 153
    see also free market; internal market;
        privatisation; quasi-markets
Marxism and Marxist perspectives
    contradictory position of welfare
        state 15
    critiques of the professions 87–8
    linked with collectivism 67
    Marxist-feminism 34–5
    on society make-up 33
    theory 33–4
    on welfare state development 13–14
mediated professional power 88
medical model of health care, alternative
    consciousness approach 27
medical power 27
    effect of purchaser/provider
        reforms 102
    NHS concessions to 95
    see also professional power
Mental Health Act 1959 60
mental health services, status 61
Mental Treatment Act 1930 54
Metropolitan Poor Act 1867 75
midwifery services 54
Midwives Act 1902 94
minimal state model of health care 48,
    78
    compatible with individualism 67
monetarism 112
monopolists, professional 35–6, 37
mutual aid associations 76–7
    see also Friendly Societies

National Health Insurance
    (NHI) 51–2, 55, 75
    politics of 52–3
National Health Service (NHS)
    bureaucracy increasing 99–100, 104,
        106
    commitment to individual rights 75
    consumer choice 117–18, 120, 126–7
    costs 8, 60–1, 69–70, 78
    effect of level of social care on 17

founding principles 4, 19
fragmentation of? 165
funding, post-war principles 4
funding alternatives 113, 115, 156
the future 182–5
inequalities in 61–2
internal differences within medical
    profession 35–6
managerial culture 43
marketising 114–18
as a monopoly 6, 8
organisational structure 62
origin of reforms 114
planning system 42–3
politics of organisation 56–9
politics of reorganisation 62–4
a professional network 39
property management 160–1
rationing of health care 123, 124
reflection of social democratic
    principles 4
reform difficulties 9
review of 114–15
Royal Commission (1979) 64–5
trusts 116, 117, 163, 164
see also Beveridge Report; health care;
    managers, professional;
    quasi-markets
National Health Service and Community
    Care Act 1990 102
need 118–24
atomisation of 119–20
comparative 119
equation with economic
    matters 120–1
expressed 119
felt 119
negative definition of 123
normative 118–19
relative *v.* absolute 119–20
typology 118–19
needs, prioritisation of 141
neo-conservatism 7, 113
neo-liberalism 111
schools of thought 111–12
neo-pluralism 32–3
neo-Weberian critique of the
    professions 88–9
Netherlands 175–6, 178, 179
Dekker/Simons plan 175, 177, 182
networks *see* policy networks
New Deal 93, 105
New Managerialism 100–1

New Right perspective 6–9, 91–2,
    171–3
alternatives to state welfare 76
and consumer choice 130
economic growth belief 5
economic liberal theories 6–7
individual freedom of choice 70
and individualism 67, 68–9
neo-Conservative theories 7
solution to welfare state
    problems 8–9
v. welfare pluralist perspective 16–17
see also privatisation; Thatcherism
NHI *see* National Health Insurance
NHS *see* National Health Service
NHS trusts 116, 117, 163, 164
non-state health care 48–9
v. state health care 52, 67
Nurse Registration Act 1919 93
nurses, importance of individualism 68
nursing
history of 93–4
impact of Griffiths Report 99
'new nursing' 94
pay reviews 104–5
nursing homes, private sector 158–9,
    160

optical checkups 156
outdoor relief 49

partisan mutual adjustment (PMA) 30,
    140
Patient's Charter 68, 92, 139
postponement of operations 144
standards 144
three new rights 144
patriarchy, in medical profession 89, 90
patronage model of professional
    power 87–8
paupers 51, 54
pay levels and awards 161–2
pay reviews, nursing 104–5
performance indicators (PIs) 104, 105
pluralism 30, 31–3, 140
neo-pluralism 32–3
see also welfare pluralism
PMA (partisan mutual adjustment) 30,
    140
policy
by default 31
description 23, 24

policy (*cont.*)
  implementation in a
      quasi-market   124–7
  interpretation of   24
  methods of emergence   23, 24, 24–5
  organisational influence on   31
policy communities   39, 40
policy making
  devolution of   32–3
  difficulties of   24
  incrementalism   29–30
  information *v.* participation   24
  'muddling through'   30
  and power   25, 26–8, 30
  radical or incremental?   43–4
  rational or political?   42–3
  restriction of interest group access
      to   32
  Thatcherite   124–5
  see also decision making
policy networks   38–41
  forces for change   40
  issue networks   39–40, 140
  professional networks   39
  stability in   40
  state's role in   38, 39, 40–1
  typology of   39
  unorthodoxy in   40, 41–2
Poor Law   48, 49, 54
  hospital services   54
  infirmaries   51
  medical services   51, 74
populism   113
power
  covert   27
  distribution in society   26
  in health care   44
  personal   27
  and policy making   25, 26–8, 30
  within the state   31–5
  see also empowerment; medical power;
      professional power
power structures   87–8
prescriptions   181
  generic prescribing   181
Prevention and Health   70, 73
private acute care   159, 160
private health insurance 76
  expansion of   159
  tax relief   115, 124, 138, 160
privatisation   110, 112, 131
  cultural and ideological content   151
  defined   150–1

and economic growth   152
elements of   157
future of   164–7
and independence   154
individualist *v.* collectivist   151
motivations for   151–5
in practice   155–64
in theory   151–5
producer monopolies   153
professional monopolists   35–6, 37
professional power   27, 85–94
  in the 1990s   101–5
  influence on health policy   94–7
  rise of   92–4
  types of   87–8
  see also medical power
professionals
  effect of industrialisation   85
  and the public interest   32–3
  see also professional power
professional society   84
professions
  altruism?   86, 87, 89
  critical approaches to   87–92
  exclusionary closure   88–9, 89–90
  feminist critique   89–91
  functionalist approach   86–7, 87
  Marxist critiques   87–8
  neo-Weberian critique   88–9
  proliferation of groups   85–6
  semi-professions   89, 90, 94, 96
  traditional approaches to   86–7
  trait approach   86, 87
proletarianisation   88
property management, NHS   160–1
providers   102, 116, 120, 121, 126
  as flexible firms   162–4
  influence of   44
  trusts   117
proxy consumers   139
public expenditure, categories   14
public health medicine   121–3
purchasers   102, 116–17, 121, 126
  GP fundholders as   139
  and the private sector   116

quality assurance
  Germany   180
  Netherlands   179
  see also standards
quasi-markets   113, 115–18, 120–1, 163,
    173
  policy implementation in   124–7

racial discrimination in medicine 134–5
racism 18
  levels of operation of 19
radical feminism 11, 34
rationalisers, corporate 35, 36
rationality, in decision making 28–9
'rational planning' 59–60
rationing, of health care 123, 124
Redcliffe-Maud Commission 63
Regional Health Authorities
  (RHAs) 63
residential homes, private sector 158–9,
  160
residual model of state welfare *see*
  minimal state model
resource allocation 42–3
  inequalities 61–2
Resource Allocation Working Party 72
Resource Management Initiative 103
RHAs (Regional Health
  Authorities) 63
rights 74–81
  to health care 67–8
  NHS commitment to 75
  Patient's Charter 144
Royal Commission (1979) 64–5

Salmon Report 93–4
Sanitary Act 1866 50
Second Green Paper 63, 64
Seebohm Committee 63
selectivity 78–81
  disadvantages of 79–81
self-help, through privatisation 154
self-help therapies 92
semi-professions 89, 90, 94, 96
sexual harassment 89
Simons Plan (Netherlands) 175, 177,
  182
social capital 14, 15
social care costs, *v*. NHS costs 126
social democratic perspective 2, 2–6
  aim 2–3
  combatting inequalities 3, 5
  compatible with collectivism 67
  principles reflected in National Health
    Service 4
  Second World War and after 3
social expenses 14, 15
social insurance model of health
  care 51, 56
socialist feminists 10–11
social policy reforms, post-war 59

Social Services Committee enquiry 162
Social Services Departments 63
standard operating procedures
  (SOPs) 31
standards 179
  Patient's Charter 144
  see also quality assurance
state intervention 152
state *v*. non-state health care roles 52,
  67
state welfare, alternatives to 76
Stockholm Syndrome 144
support workers 105
Sweden 177–8, 179, 180, 182

tax, for funding the NHS? 142
tax relief, private health insurance 115,
  124, 138, 160
teaching hospitals, status within
  NHS 58–9
tendering, competitive 154, 155, 166
  for ancillary services 161
Thatcherism 111–13
  policy making 124–5
theology *v*. medicine 85
Thomlinson Report 100
trusts 116, 117, 163, 164
two nations perspective 154

United States of America
  (USA) 176–7, 179, 180
  Clinton proposals 176–7, 178
  Diagnostic Related Groups 179
  insurance 132, 176
  Medicare and Medicaid
    programmes 176
universalism 19, 55–6
universalist/citizenship model 59–62,
  65
  compatible with collectivism 67
  costs affordable? 78
  movement towards 53–6
urbanisation 49–50
USA *see* United States of America
user groups 141, 142

voluntary sector
  associations 76–7
  and the chronically sick 50
  hospitals 49, 50, 54–5, 57, 77
  see also Friendly Societies
vouchers, NHS 115

wage levels and awards   161–2
waiting lists   134
Weber   *see* neo-Weberian critique
welfare
  alternatives to state provision   76
  mixed economy of   *see* welfare
    pluralism
welfare bureaucracies   130, 131
welfare pluralism and
    perspectives   15–17, 151, 152, 172
  and collectivism   67, 74
  v. New Right perspective   16–17
  in NHS organisation   53
welfare policies, and economic
    growth   5–6
welfare schemes, employer-based   76
welfare state
  Marxist views   13–14, 15
  problems and solutions, New Right
    views   8

Willink Plan   57
Wilson Committee   145
women
  discrimination in medical school
    admissions   134
  doctors' view of   11–12
  domestic role   10–11
  marginalisation of   90–1
  power of medical profession over   90
  professional exclusion and
    demarcation   89–90
  unequal social position   90
  as users and providers of health
    care   10, 12
workhouse test   48
Working for Patients   124, 125, 137–8,
    173
World Health Organisation
  Alma Ata declaration   133–4
  Healthy Cities approach   74